Ancient Chinese Weapons

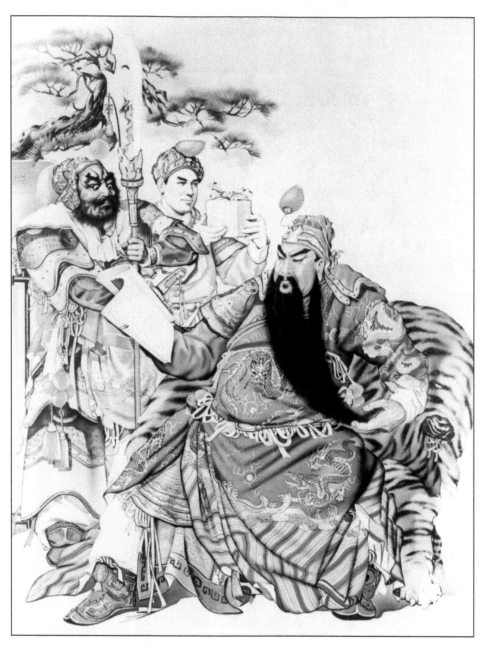

General Guan Yu, Three Kingdoms Period

Ancient Chinese Weapons
A Martial Artist's Guide

中國古代兵器

Dr. Yang, Jwing-Ming

楊俊敏博士

Text illustrations by
Marc Mannheimer and Scott Johnston

YMAA Publication Center
Wolfeboro, NH USA

YMAA Publication Center
Main Office:
    PO Box 480
    Wolfeboro, NH 03894
    800-669-8892 • info@ymaa.com • www.ymaa.com

Publisher's Cataloging in Publication
(Prepared by Quality Books Inc.)

Yang, Jwing-Ming, 1946-
        Ancient chinese weapons : a martial artist's
    guide / Yang Jwing-Ming. -- 1st ed.
        p. cm.
        Includes index.
        ISBN: 1-886969-67-1

        1. Martial arts weapons--China.   I. Title.

GV1101.5.Y36 1999   796.8'15'028
                                    QBI98-1725

20200302

Text illustrations by Marc Mannheimer and Scott Johnston
Cover illustration by Marc Mannheimer
Cover design by Richard Rossiter

ISBN: 9781886969674

Printed in USA

Dedicated to my Long Fist Grandmaster
Han, Ching-Tang
謹奉獻給韓慶堂老師

Romanization of Chinese Words

This book uses the Pinyin romanization system of Chinese to English. Pinyin is standard in the People's Republic of China, and in several world organizations, including the United Nations. Pinyin, which was introduced in China in the 1950's, replaces the Wade-Giles and Yale systems. In some cases, the more popular spelling of a word may be used for clarity.

Some common conversions:

Pinyin	Also Spelled As	Pronunciation
Qi	Chi	chē
Qigong	Chi Kung	chē kǔng
Qin Na	Chin Na	chǐn nǎ
Jin	Jing	jǐn
Gongfu	Kung Fu	gōng foo
Taijiquan	Tai Chi Chuan	tī jē chüén

For more information, please refer to *The People's Republic of China: Administrative Atlas, The Reform of the Chinese Written Language,* or a contemporary manual of style.

Contents

About the Author

Yang, Jwing-Ming, Ph.D., 楊俊敏博士

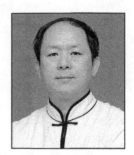

Dr. Yang, Jwing-Ming was born on August 11, 1946, in Xinzhu Xian (新竹縣), Taiwan (台灣), Republic of China (中華民國). He started his Wushu (武術) (Gongfu or Kung Fu, 功夫) training at the age of fifteen under the Shaolin White Crane (少林白鶴) Master Cheng, Gin-Gsao (曾金灶). Master Cheng originally learned Taizuquan (太祖拳) from his grandfather when he was a child. When Master Cheng was fifteen years old, he started learning White Crane from Master Jin, Shao-Feng (金紹峰), and followed him for twenty-three years until Master Jin's death.

In thirteen years of study (1961-1974) under Master Cheng, Dr. Yang became an expert in the White Crane Style of Chinese martial arts, which includes both the use of barehands and of various weapons such as saber, staff, spear, trident, two short rods, and many other weapons. With the same master he also studied White Crane Qigong (氣功), Qin Na (or Chin Na, 擒拿), Tui Na (推拿) and Dian Xue massages (點穴按摩), and herbal treatment.

At the age of sixteen, Dr. Yang began the study of Yang Style Taijiquan (楊氏太極拳) under Master Kao Tao (高濤). After learning from Master Kao, Dr. Yang continued his study and research of Taijiquan with several masters and senior practitioners such as Master Li, Mao-Ching (李茂清) and Mr. Wilson Chen (陳威伸) in Taipei (台北). Master Li learned his Taijiquan from the well-known Master Han, Ching-Tang (韓慶堂), and Mr. Chen learned his Taijiquan from Master Zhang, Xiang-San (張祥三). Dr. Yang has mastered the Taiji barehand sequence, pushing hands, the two-man fighting sequence, Taiji sword, Taiji saber, and Taiji Qigong.

When Dr. Yang was eighteen years old he entered Tamkang College (淡江學院) in Taipei Xian to study Physics. In college he began the study of traditional Shaolin Long Fist (Changquan or Chang Chuan, 少林長拳) with Master Li, Mao-Ching at the Tamkang College Guoshu Club (淡江國術社) (1964-1968), and eventually became an assistant instructor under Master Li. In 1971 he completed his M.S. degree in Physics at the National Taiwan University (台灣大學), and then served in the Chinese Air Force from 1971 to 1972. In the service, Dr. Yang taught Physics at the Junior Academy of the Chinese Air Force (空軍幼校) while also teaching Wushu. After being honorably discharged in 1972, he returned to Tamkang College to teach Physics and resumed study under Master Li, Mao-Ching. From Master Li, Dr. Yang learned Northern Style Wushu, which includes both barehand (especially kicking) techniques and numerous weapons.

In 1974, Dr. Yang came to the United States to study Mechanical Engineering at Purdue University. At the request of a few students, Dr. Yang began to teach Gongfu (Kung Fu), which resulted in the foundation of the Purdue University Chinese Kung Fu Research Club in the spring of 1975. While at Purdue, Dr. Yang also taught college-credited courses in Taijiquan. In May of 1978 he was awarded a Ph.D. in Mechanical Engineering by Purdue.

In 1980, Dr. Yang moved to Houston to work for Texas Instruments. While in Houston he founded Yang's Shaolin Kung Fu Academy, which was eventually taken over by his disciple Mr. Jeffery Bolt, after Dr. Yang moved to Boston in 1982. Dr. Yang founded Yang's Martial Arts Academy (YMAA) in Boston on October 1, 1982.

In January of 1984 he gave up his engineering career to devote more time to research, writing, and teaching. In March of 1986 he purchased property in the Jamaica Plain area of Boston to be used as the headquarters of the new organization, Yang's Martial Arts Association. The organization has continued to expand, and, as of July 1, 1989, YMAA has become just one division of Yang's Oriental Arts Association, Inc. (YOAA, Inc.).

In summary, Dr. Yang has been involved in Chinese Wushu since 1961. During this time, he has spent thirteen years learning Shaolin White Crane (Bai He), Shaolin Long Fist (Changquan), and Taijiquan. Dr. Yang has more than thirty years of instructional experience: seven years in Taiwan, five years at Purdue University, two years in Houston, Texas, and sixteen years in Boston, Massachusetts.

In addition, Dr. Yang has been invited to offer seminars around the world to share his knowledge of Chinese martial arts and Qigong. The countries he has visited include Canada, Mexico, France, Italy, Poland, England, Ireland, Portugal, Switzerland, Germany, Hungary, Spain, Holland, Belgium, Latvia, South Africa, Morocco, Iran, Venezuela, Chile, Bermuda, Barbados, and Saudi Arabia.

Since 1986, YMAA has become an international organization, which currently includes forty-four schools located in Poland, Portugal, France, Italy, Holland, Hungary, South America, Ireland, Belgium, the United Kingdom, Chile, Venezuela, Canada, and the United States. Many of Dr. Yang's books and videotapes have been translated into languages such as French, Italian, Spanish, Polish, Czech, Bulgarian, Russian, Hungarian, and Farsi.

Dr. Yang has published twenty-two other volumes on the martial arts and Qigong:

1. *Shaolin Chin Na;* Unique Publications, Inc., 1980.
2. *Shaolin Long Fist Kung Fu;* Unique Publications, Inc., 1981.
3. *Yang Style Tai Chi Chuan;* Unique Publications, Inc., 1981.
4. *Introduction to Ancient Chinese Weapons;* Unique Publications, Inc., 1985.

5. *Qigong—Health and Martial Arts;* YMAA Publication Center, 1985.

6. *Northern Shaolin Sword;* YMAA Publication Center, 1985.

7. *Tai Chi Theory and Martial Power;* YMAA Publication Center, 1986.

8. *Tai Chi Chuan Martial Applications,* YMAA Publication Center, 1986.

9. *Analysis of Shaolin Chin Na;* YMAA Publication Center, 1987.

10. *Eight Simple Qigong Exercises for Health;* YMAA Publication Center, 1988.

11. *The Root of Chinese Qigong—The Secrets of Qigong Training;* YMAA Publication Center, 1989.

12. *Muscle/Tendon Changing and Marrow/Brain Washing Chi Kung—The Secret of Youth;* YMAA Publication Center, 1989.

13. *Hsing Yi Chuan—Theory and Applications;* YMAA Publication Center, 1990.

14. *The Essence of Taiji Qigong—The Internal Foundation of Taijiquan;* YMAA Publication Center, 1990.

15. *Qigong for Arthritis;* YMAA Publication Center, 1991.

16. *Chinese Qigong Massage—General Massage;* YMAA Publication Center, 1992.

17. *How to Defend Yourself;* YMAA Publication Center, 1992.

18. *Baguazhang—Emei Baguazhang;* YMAA Publication Center, 1994.

19. *Comprehensive Applications of Shaolin Chin Na—The Practical Defense of Chinese Seizing Arts;* YMAA Publication Center, 1995.

20. *Taiji Chin Na—The Seizing Art of Taijiquan;* YMAA Publication Center, 1995.

21. *The Essence of Shaolin White Crane;* YMAA Publication Center, 1996.

22. *Back Pain—Chinese Qigong for Healing and Prevention;* YMAA Publication Center, 1997.

Dr. Yang has also published the following videotapes:

1. *Yang Style Tai Chi Chuan and Its Applications;* YMAA Publication Center, 1984.

2. *Shaolin Long Fist Kung Fu—Lien Bu Chuan and Its Applications;* YMAA Publication Center, 1985.

3. *Shaolin Long Fist Kung Fu—Gung Li Chuan and Its Applications;* YMAA Publication Center, 1986.

4. *Shaolin Chin Na;* YMAA Publication Center, 1987.

5. *Wai Dan Chi Kung, Vol. 1—The Eight Pieces of Brocade;* YMAA Publication Center, 1987.

6. *Chi Kung for Tai Chi Chuan;* YMAA Publication Center, 1990.

7. *Qigong for Arthritis;* YMAA Publication Center, 1991.

8. *Qigong Massage—Self Massage;* YMAA Publication Center, 1992.

9. *Qigong Massage—With a Partner;* YMAA Publication Center, 1992.

10. *Defend Yourself 1—Unarmed Attack;* YMAA Publication Center, 1992.

11. *Defend Yourself 2—Knife Attack;* YMAA Publication Center, 1992.

12. *Comprehensive Applications of Shaolin Chin Na 1;* YMAA Publication Center, 1995.

13. *Comprehensive Applications of Shaolin Chin Na 2;* YMAA Publication Center, 1995.

14. *Shaolin Long Fist Kung Fu—Yi Lu Mai Fu & Er Lu Mai Fu;* YMAA Publication Center, 1995.

15. *Shaolin Long Fist Kung Fu—Shi Zi Tang;* YMAA Publication Center, 1995.

16. *Taiji Chin Na;* YMAA Publication Center, 1995.

17. *Emei Baguazhang—1;* Basic Training, Qigong, Eight Palms, and Applications; YMAA Publication Center, 1995.

18. *Emei Baguazhang—2;* Swimming Body Baguazhang and Its Applications; YMAA Publication Center, 1995.

19. *Emei Baguazhang—3;* Bagua Deer Hook Sword and Its Applications YMAA Publication Center, 1995.

20. *Xingyiquan—12 Animal Patterns and Their Applications;* YMAA Publication Center, 1995.

21. *24 and 48 Simplified Taijiquan;* YMAA Publication Center, 1995.

22. *White Crane Hard Qigong;* YMAA Publication Center, 1997.

23. *White Crane Soft Qigong;* YMAA Publication Center, 1997.

24. *Xiao Hu Yan—Intermediate Level Long Fist Sequence;* YMAA Publication Center, 1997.

25. *Back Pain—Chinese Qigong for Healing and Prevention;* YMAA Publication Center, 1997.

26. *Scientific Foundation of Chinese Qigong;* YMAA Publication Center, 1997.

27. *Taijiquan—Classical Yang Style;* YMAA Publication Center, 1999.

28. *Taiji Sword and Applications—Classical Yang Style;* YMAA Publication Center, 1999.

Foreword

Jeff Bolt

It is well-known that the Chinese martial arts have a very rich history and contain many different styles. These styles can be divided into two general categories; internal and external. These categories can further be divided into more sub-categories and systems, either by geographic location, family systems, religious orientation and others. Even though the many styles and systems of the Chinese martial arts are diverse, they all utilized the same weapons that were available at that time in their history.

In the study of Chinese Martial arts, it is important that the practitioner also have an understanding of the history of their art. Some styles practiced techniques that were restricted, or determined by the clothes worn at that time of the style's development. Some emphasized techniques needed for close quarters, while others were not restricted by space. Those styles, presumably, can be expanded upon or modified slightly for the clothing worn today, or because of less restrictions on space, without diverting from the essence of the style itself.

Likewise, many styles utilized various weapons that were available. Many weapons were simple farm tools and instruments, which depended upon the type of crops or livestock that was prevalent in that area of the country. It is also important to understand this history, so that one does not "restrict" the practice of one's art to only those techniques or weapons that were used under different historical circumstances.

In this book, Dr. Yang provides an invaluable view of the many weapons used throughout Chinese martial arts history. This will help the practitioner and enthusiast to better understand the reasons why their particular style uses the weapons that they do.

I am especially honored to write the foreword for this book. Master Yang has been my teacher since he first came to the United States from Taiwan in 1974. I began my training under Master Yang in January of 1975, while a student at Purdue University. He has been a teacher, a father and a friend. Learning from Master Yang is never-ending, since he himself continues to learn, research and practice the Chinese martial arts to their full potential. The only limitations to an individual's capability in the martial arts are their own lack of vision, perseverance, and dedication. Master Yang has shown us all that he suffers from none of these afflictions.

Jeff Bolt
August, 1998

Preface

Since 1973, when President Nixon opened the gate to Communist China, the cultural exchange between the East and the West has greatly influenced both societies. Chinese cultural treasures, such as acupuncture, martial arts, Qigong, painting, music, calligraphy, Confucianism, Daoism, and Buddhism are no longer strange concepts to Westerners. In order to expedite this cultural exchange, in 1984 I resigned my engineering job and put all my effort into translating classics of Chinese culture into Western languages. Through seminars, instruction, and publication, I have attempted to incorporate Chinese wisdom of the ages into our hurried, modern world. Unfortunately, all my effort has been limited to the knowledge of my own personal experience. The exchange in many other fields is still waiting for the expertise of other qualified contributors.

The fields which with I am most familiar are Chinese martial arts and Qigong. After thirteen years of effort, I have published twenty-two books and twenty-five videotapes. Many of these publications have also been translated into other languages. YMAA (Yang's Martial Arts Association) was originally founded under this charter. Today, YMAA Publication Center publishes not only my writings, but also those of many other authors involved in the exploration of Oriental culture. Moreover, YMAA schools have multiplied from only a few, just thirteen years ago, to now more than forty, in no less than fourteen different countries.

During this time of great cultural exchange, I am convinced that the authoritative information which we can provide to the public is critical in order to help the seeker filter out useless, exploitative fantasy, and direct them on to the path of true understanding. For example, due to a lack of profound publications regarding the philosophy of Chinese martial arts, most Westerners still believe the main goal of Chinese martial arts training is fighting, rather than spiritual cultivation. Moreover, many so called "psychic Qigong masters" in China have contributed to a misunderstanding of Qigong, and have cast its practice in an unfavorable light, with their wild and insupportable claims of miraculous healing through their own "psychic" powers. These frauds serve only to bring increased suffering into the world for their own financial gain. They have also delayed true scientific verification and acceptance of ancient Chinese Qigong by Western medical practitioners.

In order to provide a clear understanding of Chinese martial arts, I wrote the book, *Introduction to Ancient Chinese Weapons,* published in 1985 by Unique Publications. However, due to a lack of information at that time, the contents of the book were not as thorough as I originally wished. Now, there is more information available. Therefore, I believe that the time has come to update the original book. Naturally, this new book should not be considered the final authority in this field. There have simply been too many weapon developments and refinements over the more than seven thousand years of Chinese history for any one book to cover. What this book can provide you with is an historical overview of weapon concepts and trends for your study and enjoyment.

Due to lack of information, great battle engines such as siege machines, troop carriers, firearms, fortification defenses, battering rams, and catapults are not covered in this book. This book instead will focus on squad level weapons which were carried by Chinese martial artists and soldiers. I sincerely hope to someday see more knowledgeable scholars than myself publish other volumes covering the subject of these great war machines, as well as those weapons introduced in this book.

Acknowledgments

Thanks to Richard Rossiter for his cover design and Tim Comrie for typesetting. Thanks also to Marc Mannheimer and Scott Johnston for their drawings, to James Yang and Mei-Ling Yang, for general help, to Erik Elsemans, Chris Hartgrove, June-Marie Mahay, Chris Fazzio, Jeff Pratt, Andrew Murray, Nicholas C. Yang, and many other YMAA members for proofing the manuscript and for contributing many valuable suggestions and discussions. Special thanks to James O'Leary for his editing.

CHAPTER 1

General Introduction

一般介紹

1-1. INTRODUCTION

Chinese Wushu (武術) (martial techniques), known to Westerners as martial arts, has evolved in China for over 5,000 years. This evolution has been experienced not only by the many schools of barehand fighting, but also by a wide variety of weapons practitioners. As various types of weaponry have evolved, so have the materials and techniques for their fabrication. From the most primitive weapons made of stone, one can trace their development through copper, brass, iron and finally very strong yet light alloys.

Although the art of Chinese weapons mastery has enjoyed a glorious past, its future remains doubtful. Modern culture leads people away from the study of ancient weapons for a variety of reasons. First, guns, with their ease of operation and greater killing potential, have made people believe that understanding martial weapons is impractical. Second, very few qualified masters are around to teach, and thereby preserve, the artistry of handling ancient weapons. Finally, becoming proficient in any martial art (especially those involving weaponry) requires much time, patience and practice. In today's society, few people appear willing to exert the energy necessary for learning the ancient art of Chinese weapons.

The study and practice of Chinese weapons, like that of any martial art, has value far beyond that derived from perfecting the techniques. There is an intrinsic historical value. This art form has been developing for over 5,000 years, it represents an incredible evolution of human culture. There is also the more conventional artistic value. Like a fine dancer, the martial artist exhibits total control of his or her body. There is value for one's health. Perfecting the art of Chinese weapons requires extensive physical training, which enables the entire body to become strong and well-conditioned. Of course, there is the personal self-defense value. Martial weapons originated for defensive purposes. Practicing with them trains one's perception and reaction time, allowing for quick and correct maneuvering. Moral value remains the most important aspect

1

of the art of martial weapons. The practitioner must learn patience, perseverance and humility. With diligence and dedication, one will strengthen his spiritual confidence and power.

By their sheer numbers, ancient Chinese weapons confuse most martial artists. Adding to this confusion is the fact that many weapons developed in places other than China. For classification purposes, Oriental weapons commonly used today are: Chinese, Japanese, Korean, Indochinese, and Okinawan types.

Almost all Oriental weapons originated in China and were subsequently exported to other cultures. Following centuries of evolution in different cultures, the weapons necessarily became dissimilar. Hopefully, this book will clarify the confusion that these circumstances have created.

1-2. COMMON KNOWLEDGE

In ancient China, weapons varied greatly. These variations arose from differences in: 1) the terrain from one province to another; 2) physical traits of martial artists; 3) local culture and lifestyles; and 4) the special purposes of each weapon. To be a knowledgeable martial artist, one must understand these differences in addition to knowing the Chinese weapons themselves. Therefore, this section will discuss the classification of Chinese weapons and will explain the relationships between weapons and Chinese geography, martial artists and fighting strategy.

Classification of Chinese Weapons. At one time, the Chinese word for "weapons" was Bingqi (兵器) which translates into "soldier instruments." Later, it was shortened to just Bing (兵). Thus, Chang Bing (長兵) means "long weapons" and Duan Bing (短兵) means "short weapons." Another term commonly used by Chinese is Wuqi (武器) which literally translates as "martial instruments" or "martial weapons."

During the 5,000 year history of Bingqi (兵器), styles, shapes, materials and fabrication techniques have changed from one dynasty to the next. Within the period of one dynasty, some of which have lasted 800 years, countless numbers of Chinese weapons evolved.

To characterize this multitude of arms, eighteen kinds of weapons including long, short, very short, soft and projectile were chosen. A martial artist proficient with all of these types wassaid to have mastered the Shi Ba Ban Wuyi (十八般武藝) or "eighteen kinds of martial techniques."

In this section, the "eighteen" representative weapons, chosen for three different eras, are listed. The common weapons classified as long, short, soft, and projectile and thrown will be listed in Appendix A, which will include the Chinese spelling, pronunciation and English translation.

Table 1-1. Eighteen Representative Weapons.
(Shi Ba Ban Wu Qi)
十八般武器

Spring and Autumn Period and Warring States Period (772-222 B.C.)	Han Dynasty (206 B.C.-220 A.D.)	Song Dynasty (960-1280 A.D.)
	Spear (Qiang- 槍)	
	Halberd (Ji- 戟)	
Long Rod (Gun- 棍)		
Iron Bar (Tie- 鐵)		
	Trident (Cha- 叉)	
Horse Fork (Tang- 鎲)		
	Hook (Gou- 鉤)	
Eighteen-Chi Tapered Rod (Shuo- 槊)		
Ring (Huan- 環)		
	Saber (Dao- 刀)	
	Sword (Jian- 劍)	
Crutches (Guai- 柺)		
	Axe (Fu- 斧)	
	Whip (Bian- 鞭)	
	Sai (Jian- 鐧 or Chai- 釵)	
	Hammer (Chui- 錘)	
	Short Staff or Club (Bang- 棒)	
Pestle (Chu- 杵)		
	Bow and Arrow (Gong Jian- 弓箭)	
	Long-Handled Battle Axe (Yue- 鉞)	
	Long-Handled Claw (Zhua- 抓)	
	Sickle (Lian- 鐮)	
Piercing Spear (Jue- 鈌)		
Battle Strategy (Bing Fa- 兵法)		
		Cross Bow (Nu- 弩)
		Lance (Mao- 矛)
		Shield (Dun- 盾)
		Harrow, Rake (Ba- 鈀)
		Flat-Head Halberd (Ge- 戈)

Problems arise in trying to present a relatively simple classification of Chinese weapons. First, the same weapon can have a different name in different dynasties, e.g., Shu (殳) (twelve-chi tapered rod) in the Han Dynasty (206-220 B.C., 漢朝) is identical to Zhang Er (丈二) in the Qing Dynasty (1644-1911 A.D., 清朝). Second, a weapon with a very minor design change often received a new name. The flat-headed halberd of the Shang Dynasty(1751-1111 B.C., 商朝) was called Ge (戈), but the sharp-headed, yet otherwise identical halberd of Spring and Autumn Period and Warring States Period (722-222 B.C., 春秋戰國) was called the Ji (戟). Finally, many weapons are known from history but their exact structures remain mysteries. For example, the Fa (法) of the Han Dynasty (201 B.C.-220 A.D., 漢朝) was considered one of the eighteen weapons; but Fa probably meant "battle strategy" rather than an actual weapon. Jue (鈌) was some kind of spear-like piercing weapon, but it does not exist today. Huan (環) translates as "ring," but it belongs in the class of long weapons. Ben (錛), which derived from the tool "adze," was used by carpenters, but the details of its structure remain unclear.

1-3. WEAPONS AND CHINESE GEOGRAPHY

A country as vast as China encompasses many types of terrain. Whereas deserts and high plateaus cover the northern territory, mountain ranges dominate the west. The southeast coast and central zones, favored by the Chinese for thousands of years, are lush and warm with many lakes, ponds and rivers.

These geographic distinctions produced significant differences in the evolution of local cultures. Physical traits as well as ethnic traditions varied from area to area. Such differences caused variations in the weapons that developed. For example, Northern Chinese tend to be taller and more powerful than their southern brethren. Martial artists from the north utilized longer and heavier weapons. On the contrary, Southern Chinese, being shorter and generally weaker, would adopt shorter and lighter weapons appropriate for their stature. As an example, the long rod normally carried by southern martial artists was at least half a foot shorter than that of its northern counterpart.

Cultural backgrounds and the resulting lifestyles in different areas contributed to variations in weaponry. Northern China, because of the wide expanse of countryside, developed a culture very similar to that of Texas and the old west in North America. These people were more wild and much better at fighting on horse back than those from the south. Southern Chinese martial artists were more of a cosmopolitan type, who lived in a more crowded environment and grew to become better at ground fighting. Also, because of the warmer weather and wide spread bodies of water in the south, southern people were generally better at swimming and fighting in the water than northern inhabitants.

Distinctions existed also between people of the west and southeast. Because of the mountains in the west, the local people specialized in hunting with a trident. Naturally, they often used the same weapon when fighting. Also, poisonous animals such as snakes, spiders, and centipedes were common in the western mountains. After thousands of years of experience, people learned how to deal with these poisons. This special knowledge made western martial artists expert in utilizing poison on their weapons to kill an enemy more easily. The southeast, unlike the west, was a great agricultural plain. People used the hoe and harrow for cultivation. As a result, hoe and harrow fighting techniques developed.

Furthermore, the country was so vast that in ancient times the central government exerted little control in the areas distant from the capital. During harvest season, large groups of bandits would swoop down and rob entire villages. To combat such attacks, a village would hire a martial artist to teach the young people defense. Because the bandits struck with little warning, the defenders used whatever was at hand as a weapon. Therefore, the people became adept with the hoe, rake, harrow, trident, or other common farming or hunting tools as weapons of defense.

With time, communication and transportation improved throughout China. As weapons spread around the country, local distinctions were lost and martial styles and techniques became a national mixture.

1-4. WEAPONS AND MARTIAL ARTISTS

Generally speaking, a well-trained martial artist would carry at least three kinds of weapons. He would have a primary weapon such as a sword, saber, staff, or spear, with which he was most proficient. Usually this weapon was obvious to his enemy and had the most power and killing potential. A secondary weapon would be hidden on his body, perhaps a whip or an iron chain in his belt or a pair of daggers in his boots, which could be used in the event that his main weapon was lost during battle. For use at very long distances or in a surprise attack in a close battle, he would use dart weapons. Some of these easily-hidden weapons (e.g., darts or throwing knives) were thrown by hand, others (e.g., needles) were spat from the mouth, and still others (e.g., sleeve arrows) were projected from a spring-equipped tube.

In choosing his weapons, a martial artist must consider three factors. First, what weapon suits his physical stature? If he is tall and strong, he would take advantage of a long, heavy weapon such as a large saber or halberd, which may weigh over 50 pounds. These weapons have more killing potential because of their length and are more difficult to block because of their great weight.

If a martial artist is tall but not particularly strong, he might choose a spear. With this long but lighter weapon, he can effectively utilize his speed and realize greater endurance in battle. A short but very strong man might select a thick, heavy saber or a pair of hammers. Such weapons can devastate an opponent at close range.

Finally, a short and weak martial artist can best utilize swords, double swords, double sabers, double rods, or daggers. Most female Chinese martial artists specialize in these weapons.

The second factor a martial artist must consider when choosing a weapon is the conditions of an upcoming battle. Will he be on horseback facing a similarly mounted opponent? Will he be grounded but his enemy on horseback? Or, will it be a purely man-against-man encounter with no interfering steeds? Each situation requires a different weapon.

If fighting horse-to-horse, a martial artist must consider four things: protecting himself, protecting his horse, attacking his enemy, and attacking his enemy's horse. The reason for protecting himself is obvious. Protecting his horse is almost as important. He remains on equal footing with his adversary only while he is mounted. If the horse becomes disabled or the enemy knocks him off the horse, he is lost. Of course, attacking the enemy is uppermost in his mind. A long weapon such as a long staff, spear, or halberd fulfills all these requirements.

A martial artist on foot, fighting a mounted opponent, requires different weapons. His objective, killing the enemy, can be accomplished more easily if he can force him off the horse. In accomplishing that goal, a hooked sword can be used most effectively in attacking the horse's legs. Alternatively, he may use a very long, tapered rod to knock his adversary to the ground.

The final factor a martial artist considers when choosing a weapon is his own martial style. Certain weapons lend themselves better to one school than to another. For instance, Shaolin (少林) disciples were apt to use a long rod or spear, whereas Taiji practitioners more often chose the sword.

Religion too, played a role in the development of weapons in China. Monks invented weapons that had little killing potential but were still effective for self-defense, or even as tools. Their weapons often served to clear away brush as they traveled the countryside. They were also used much like a hobo's stick to carry belongings and to use as a walking stick.

During the Han (206 B.C.-220 A.D., 漢朝) and Tang (618-907 A.D., 唐朝) Dynasties, Buddhism was very popular. The Han and Tang emperors were all sincere Buddhists. In that era, many weapons were imported from Tibet, which was a stronghold of Buddhism. In the Liang Dynasty (502-557 A.D., 梁朝), priests became more involved with weapons and by the time of the Song Dynasty (960-1280 A.D., 宋), Shaolin priests were active martial artists perfecting deadly techniques.

To be able to effectively utilize various weapons on different occasions, a martial artist would practice and specialize in at least one long weapon and one short weapon. Because the main principles within each class of weapons are the same, it would be simple for a well-trained martial artist to effectively utilize any weapon instantly. Long weapon training traditionally started with the long rod, whereas short weapon training began with the saber. There is an old saying, "the long rod is the root of all the long weapons, and the saber is the pioneer of the short weapons" which implies that the long rod and the saber serve as the foundation for further work within each group of weapons. In Chinese martial society, it is said "The spear is the king of the long weapons and the sword is the leader of the short weapons."[1] This saying implies that the spear and the sword are the hardest of the long and short weapons to learn. Once a martial artist could skillfully apply them in battle, he could take advantage of the techniques and skills which the spear and sword offer. There is another proverb, "Hundred days of barehand training, thousand days of spear training, and ten thousand days of sword training."[2] From this proverb, one learns that the sword is the hardest weapon to learn. The sword is light and requires more than ten years of "internal power" training before one masters techniques for blocking heavy weapons. In addition, because the sword is usually double-edged, more technique and practice are required to effectively use both edges without dulling them. Therefore, it is said, "The sword utilizes speed and technique; the saber requires cunning, trickery, and power."[3] It is also said, "Saber, power, won by strength; sword, soft, won by technique."[4] To summarize, one can say, "The saber is like a fierce tiger; the sword is like a flying phoenix; and the spear is like a swift dragon."[5]

1-5. WEAPONS AND FIGHTING STRATEGY

Fighting strategy, a decisive factor in both large battles and personal efforts, has maintained an inseparable relationship with weapons. Some of these weapons were invented for a new battle strategy. For example, the hooked sword, together with the shield, was designed specifically for attacking horses' legs during a large battle in the Southern Song Dynasty (1127-1280 A.D., 南宋). The multi-sectional staff was created specifically for use against an enemy carrying a shield.

In the following discussion, strategies and weapons for large battles will be explained first. This type of fighting occurred in wide, open areas and included mounted cavalry and chariots. The discussion will then focus on personal battles which occurred within large battles surrounded by other warriors or on the streets of a city or in a small room.

In ancient times, large stones heaved by catapults were often the first weapons used in great battles. These very long range projectiles could kill unprotected enemies before initial man-to-man contact. The primary application of extra long-range weapons, however, was to slow down the fast-advancing cavalry.

After the invention of gunpowder, rocket arrows replaced catapulted stones as the first weapon of warfare. Not only were these arrows capable of being fired further, but they could also be rigged to explode on contact, scaring the horses and tumbling the riders to the ground. By the seventeenth and eighteenth centuries, rocket arrows had been replaced by iron balls fired from cannons.

As the enemy forces drew nearer, very long range projectiles lost effectiveness. At an intermediate distance, archers with bows and arrows could impede the enemy. As enemy forces drew even nearer, martial artists used throwing spears either from the ground, horseback, or chariots.

The battle turned into personal conflict as man fought against man. But some men might have been on horseback or in a chariot, whereas others were on foot. A very long contact weapon, such as a nine, twelve or eighteen-foot, tapered spear was effective in all three cases. A soldier on foot would often have another weapon at his disposal. To force his enemy off a horse or out of a chariot, he would often attack the horse's legs with a hooked spear while holding a greased rattan shield for protection.

Once both soldiers were on the ground, close personal fighting began. Long range weapons became less effective, so techniques and weapons shifted to the short range type.

Short range fighting in a large battle was quite different from one-on-one conflicts in a small area. The soldiers were often surrounded by others and there was no way to escape. Therefore, endurance became a key factor in determining the victor. Shorter and lighter weapons such as the sword, saber, or three sectioned staff were utilized. With hidden weapons like whips, chains, or darts, a martial artist was well prepared for a short range battle.

Some soldiers—only the very strongest—would use a long weapon even in close fighting. They had the advantage of being able to injure their enemy without exposing themselves to attack. The long staff, spear or large saber was very difficult to block because of its weight.

The martial artist using a shorter and lighter weapon emphasized speed and maneuverability when approaching the enemy. Once at close range, the long weapon which was so powerful became a hindrance to its wielder.

1-6. HISTORICAL SURVEY

History abounds with tales of terrible slaughter during the ceaseless wars that racked ancient China. These wars were fought with a vast array of martial weapons that played a major role in the development of China. From the days of stone weapons before Shen Nong (2700 B.C., 神農) to the Qing Dynasty (circa

1900 A.D., 清朝), when guns became popular, one can trace the evolution of China through the evolution of its weaponry.

The following discussion of weapons focuses on materials used in their fabrication rather than on the weapons themselves (which will be discussed in following chapters). The ancient Chinese were leaders in the metallurgical sciences. For over 3,000 years, the Chinese channeled weapons research into discovering new alloys and techniques for forging new metals which were stronger and could hold an edge better. In those days the discovery of a new alloy for sword making had as much effect on society as the discovery of atomic power in modern times.

This section will present general concepts and information concerning the evolution of Chinese martial weapons. Unfortunately, very little information exists on the entire gamut of arms. Much has been discovered about certain weapons—the narrow blade sword, for example—whereas little is known of other weapons of which only a few have been found. Because of our greater knowledge about the sword, we will focus on this weapon.

More documents have been found on the sword because the ancient Chinese considered it a more important weapon. Considered to be the highest art of Gongfu (Kung Fu), the narrow blade sword was favored by emperors, poets, and scholars alike. Confucius carried one for the noble feeling it gave him. Li, Tai Bai (李太白), a famous poet in the Tang Dynasty (618-907 A.D.) called himself "fond of drink and master of the sword."

The pure physical beauty of the sword contributed to the great appreciation it won. Mastering the complicated technique of sword fighting was so difficult that experts were held in the highest regard.

Physical beauty alone would not have been enough to account for the existence of so much more information about the sword than other weapons. The key to the preservation of the history of the sword lies in the fact that emperors and martial artists favored it. They popularized the sword to such an extent that not only did men carry them, but women, also, became attracted to them.

1-7. HISTORY AND EVOLUTION

The Chinese word for weapon, Bingqi (兵器) originated as the word for a group of weapons including the lance, spear, halberd, pronged spear, sword, and saber. Chinese people certainly used more primitive weapons than these before the advent of the language to describe them. The prehistoric Chinese, like other societies, probably utilized the sticks and stones that lay about.

Prior to Shen Nong (2700 B.C., 神農), weapons were very simple. A small stone picked up from a nearby river bed was probably the state of the art. But soon, someone discovered that a stone tied to a stick could be thrown with greater force and accuracy. Then, someone found that one stone could be used to chip and polish another to a sharp point to create a more deadly weapon. Eventually, people of this ancient society developed their first axes and spears.

Not until the time of the first recorded emperor, Huang Di (2690-2590 B.C., 黄帝), does evidence exist for advanced weapons made of material other than stone. Huang Di, called the "Yellow Emperor" because he occupied the territory near the Yellow River, had weapons made of jade, copper, and gold. This period, therefore, traditionally marks the beginning of the metallurgical sciences in arms manufacturing in China.

Knowledge of Huang Di's weapons is derived from discoveries near Zhuo Lu (涿鹿) of knives and swords—remnants of ancient battles between the Emperor's forces and those of Chi You (蚩尤). Fighting between Huang Di and Chi You also introduced the battle axe into warfare for the first time. Legend has it that Xuan Niu (玄女) (Huang Di's great-great-granddaughter) made an axe of gold engraved with a figure of a phoenix holding a sword in its mouth.

Metallurgical advances continued in China, and by the Shang Dynasty (1751-1111 B.C., 商朝), weapons made of copper alloys were in use. Bronze weapons ushered in this era, but by its close ironware had come into being.

The Zhou Dynasty (1111-1122 B.C., 周朝) replaced the Shang Dynasty following very fierce warfare. Both emperors demanded better weapons, therefore stimulating advancements in metallurgy. Emphasis, of course, was on finding alloys for stronger arms. After Zhou's victory, this emphasis changed. The years following victory were peaceful and prosperous. New metallurgical techniques were directed toward improving agricultural implements rather than arms.

As the power in the Zhou Dynasty diminished, the Emperor's control weakened and China was thrust into a series of civil wars. This time is known as the Spring and Autumn Period (722-484 B.C., 春秋) and the Warring States Period (403-222 B.C., 戰國) (Figure 1-1). Each of the many warring fac-

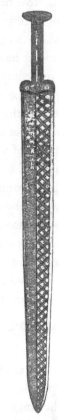

Figure 1-1. Case copper sword of King of Yue Gou Jian; discovered in 1965. Sword is 55 cm (Yue Gou Jian)(Warring States Period; 403-222 B.C.).

tions strove to produce stronger and sharper weapons. Sword makers of the day were held in the highest regard. Three of the most famous sword makers of that period were Ou Ye Zi (歐冶子), Gan Jiang (干將), and Mo Xie (莫邪).

Ou Ye Zi forged two very famous swords, Ju Que (巨闕) and Zhan Lu (湛盧). It is said that these swords were so sharp that if dipped in water they would be withdrawn perfectly dry.

Gan Jiang and Mo Xie were husband and wife. The male and female swords that they made bear their names and have a remarkable history. The legends tell how Mo Xie obtained two gold nuggets, each the size of her fist. Gan Jiang decided to forge them into a pair of swords. He built a sword oven on the top of Si Ming Mountain (四明山) in Zhejiang Province (浙江) and placed the gold inside. For three years, he heated the gold day and night but to no avail. In the fourth year, the two nuggets glowed brilliantly and rattled around the oven. Gan Jiang reasoned that the gold had not melted because no human blood had been sprinkled on it. After talking with Mo Xie, Gan Jiang prepared himself for sacrifice. He washed himself, cut his hair and fingernails, and jumped into the flaming oven. Immediately one of the nuggets melted and the Gan Jiang sword was made.

The other nugget remained solid and Mo Xie mourned for her husband. To be reunited, she leapt into the oven, the gold melted, and the Mo Xie sword was forged. The story spread quickly and Gan Jiang and Mo Xie became famous throughout China.

Of course, Mo Xie and Gan Jiang never physically threw themselves into an oven to forge their swords. The story acts as a metaphor for the great personal sacrifice that premier sword makers gave to their art. The time and energy required for forging fine weapons was all-consuming. Mo Xie and Gan Jiang may not have died for their swords, but they certainly lived for them.

The story of Mo Xie and Gan Jiang continues with the Wu emperor (吳), He Lu (闔閭), who possessed the swords and had them buried with him when he died. The swords remained hidden for 600 years. Then, in Nanchang (南昌), a scholar named Zhang Hua (張華) received a sign leading him to the swords. He witnessed a brilliant light in the sky between Tian Niu Star (天女星) and Niu Er Star (牛二星) directing him to Suzhou (蘇州), a thousand miles away. Searching in the provincial court of Suzhou, he found the Gan Jiang and Mo Xie swords at the bottom of a well in a garden.

Zhang Hua was ecstatic with his fortune and told his friend Lei Huan (雷煥). Giving him Mo Xie, he asked Lei Huan to take it to a sword maker at Luoyang (洛陽) in Henan Province (河南) to have two similar swords made. On his way to Henan, Lei Huan's boat capsized in the Yangtze River (揚子江). Both he and the Mo Xie sword were lost.

Three years later, Zhang Hua visited Loyang. Carrying the Gan Jiang sword, he traveled the very path where Mo Xie was lost. Suddenly, Gan Jiang sang out loudly. As Zhang Hua pulled out the sword, it flashed a brilliant light and leapt out of his hand into the river, thus reuniting the two swords and finishing the tale.

At the close of the Zhou Dynasty, Emperor Qin (秦) took power. The Qin Dynasty, which lasted only fifteen years (221-206 B.C.) produced no new developments in weapons. However, the Qin Dynasty is famous for the exploits of the Emperor Qin Shi (秦始皇) who was responsible for making the "Sword Pond."

Emperor Qin Shi heard tales about Wu Emperor He Lu (闔閭), who had collected tens of thousands of swords from all over China. When he died, he supposedly had the swords buried with him. Emperor Qin Shi, nearly 300 years later, wanted those weapons. He ordered his men to dig a hole in Suzhou (蘇州) where the swords were thought to be.

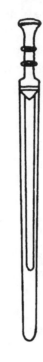

Figure 1-2. Drawing of two-foot long sword (Han Dynasty; 206-25 B.C.).

After many years of searching and digging, the Emperor had only a large hole for his efforts. Eventually, the pit filled with water and came to be known as Sword Pond (Jian Chi, 劍池).

After the Qin Dynasty came the Han Dynasty (206 B.C.-220 A.D., 漢) (Figures 1-2 and 1-3). The beginning of this era witnesses the first book about martial weapons fabrication. The book, *Huai Nan Wan Hua Shu (Huai Nan's Thousand Crafts,* 淮南萬華術*)* detailed metallurgical techniques in which the author described methods for alloying iron instead of copper to forge more progressive metal weapons than had previously been possible. The Han Dynasty also had the first contact with a foreign race. For the first time in Chinese history, people from the north and west of China entered the country in significant numbers. The ensuing conflicts produced a mixture of weapons and fighting styles.

The Three Kingdoms Dynasty followed the Han Dynasty and lasted 60 years (220-280 A.D.). The kingdoms of Cao-Cao (曹操), Liu Bei (劉備), and Sun Quan (孫權) added much to the history of martial weapons in China. King Liu Bei is known for a story about a famous sword maker of the kingdom called Pu

Yuan (蒲元), who played the key role in advancing weapons design.

The story begins with Liu Bei trying to reunite China under his rule. He occupied Shu (蜀), which today is Sichuan Province (四川省) in western China. As a descendant of the Han imperial family, he felt it was his duty to reunite China. To find the most talented men in the army, Liu Bei often presided over martial contests. One day, two men came before him in the arena. One had an iron rod, the other a long knife. As the two men fought, the rod holder gained advantage and brought the rod down toward the face of the knife wielder. To everyone's amazement, the rod snapped in two with a loud crack and sparks flew as it hit the knife.

Liu Bei stopped the fighting to ask who made the knife. "Pu Yuan"

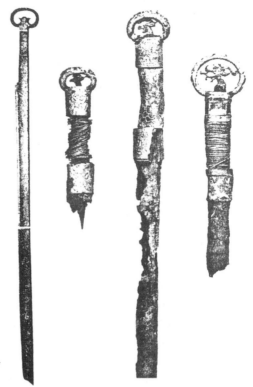

Figure 1-3. Copper narrow-blade swords (Han Dynasty; 206-25 B.C.).

came the reply. Immediately, Liu Bei sent for the gifted weapon-maker and ordered 5,000 knives for his army.

Pu Yuan was a blacksmith's son who grew up with the forge as his playmate. Helping his father shape ironware, he was already an accomplished blacksmith by his fifteenth birthday. Pu Yuan, fascinated with making blades stronger, strove day and night to find the key. One day, while holding a red-hot knife, he pondered the problem of how it could be strengthened.

For many minutes he thought with no insights and then, not realizing it had cooled, began pounding the knife. He pounded but could not shape the blade. Suddenly, inspiration struck. If the iron, which is soft when hot, hardened as it cooled slowly, would it not be harder if cooled quickly? Testing his new idea, Pu Yuan heated the blade and thrust it into cool water. When the steam lifted, he took the blade and chopped at the iron test pad. The iron pad was deeply cut, but the blade was unscathed. Pu Yuan had discovered the secret of water-quenching. He and the knife, called "miraculous knife," which "cut iron as if it were cutting mud" (削鐵如泥), became famous throughout China.

The period from the close of the Three Kingdoms to the beginning of the Liang Dynasty (梁朝) in 502 A.D. was rather unremarkable in the evolution of martial weapons. The Liang Dynasty (502-557 A.D.) marked the initiation of the Shaolin Temple's involvement in martial arts, an event that affected the development of Chinese weapons for many centuries to come. The first Shaolin Temple (少林寺) was built in 377 A.D. in Henan Province. From then until 527 A.D., the temple served as a focus of preaching and worship. Monks did not practice martial arts. In 527 A.D., Da Mo (達磨), a Buddhist prince in India, came to the temple to preach. Upon his arrival, he found that many monks were weak and sickly. To find a way to strengthen the monks, Da Mo locked himself in a cave for nine years of meditation. When he came out of the cave, he wrote his results in two books: the *Xi Sui Jing* (洗髓經) and *Yi Jin Jing* (易筋經). The former was primarily a religious treatise detailing methods for cultivating the Buddhist spirit. The latter book described methods for strengthening the body. The contents of *Xi Sui Jing* were lost after a few generations, but the Shaolin Temple taught the *Yi Jin Jing* to increase external muscular power and "internal power." With this training, Shaolin monks soon became superb martial artists.

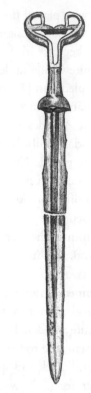

Figure 1-4. Copper, wide-blade sword (Northern Zhou Dynasty; 557-605 A.D.).

Very little is known of the weapons of the Northern Zhou Dynasty (557-581 A.D., 北周) (Figure 1-4). Apparently, copper remained the predominant metal in their fabrication. During the Sui Dynasty (581-618 A.D., 隋朝), China was united under one ruler. Local warlords vanished for a short period and the countryside remained relatively peaceful.

The Tang Dynasty (618-907 A.D., 唐朝) remains one of the brightest eras in Chinese history. A time of lasting peace, the Tang Dynasty produced many famous scholars, poets and artists. Very little effort was directed toward weapons research. In fact, the emperors of this period encouraged the people to relinquish the martial arts in favor of other, more peaceful endeavors. The Tang Dynasty ended in 907 A.D. when China was once again divided. Known as the Five

Dynasties (907-960 A.D., 五代) this period lasted only 53 years.

The Song Dynasty (960-1280 A.D., 宋朝) united China again. The most important event during the Song Dynasty occurred in 1115 A.D. when people of the Jin (金) race invaded China from Siberia, northeast of China. Prior to that time, most of the fighting in China had been internal among members of the Han race.

Invasion by the Jin precipitated development of many new weapons and martial styles. In part, this evolution resulted from the Chinese banding together to battle a common enemy. Additionally, new weapons evolved from the mixture of Chinese (Han) and Siberian (Jin) armaments.

In 1206 A.D., the Mongolians invaded China from the north. They took power and established the Yuan Dynasty (1206-1368 A.D., 元朝). This era produced many new weapons as Yuan weapons and styles mixed with those of the Han and Jin races.

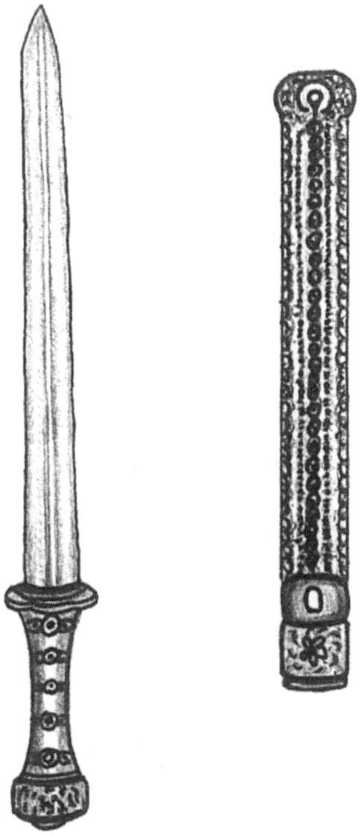

In 1368 A.D., the Han race defeated the

Figure 1-5. Narrow-blade sword used by Himalayan tribesman (Qing Dynasty; 1644-1911 A.D.).

Mongolians, and the Ming Dynasty (1368-1644 A.D., 明朝) began its long reign. An exceptionally prosperous and bright era in Chinese history, the Ming Dynasty witnessed a great expansion in the influence of Buddhism. Buddhist priests not only spread throughout China, but exported their preaching to Japan as well. With the priests went their weapons, which were adapted by the Japanese for their own use.

The Han race was once again forced from power by foreigners in 1644 A.D., this time by the Manchurians. The Manchurians formed the Qing Dynasty (1644-1911 A.D., 清朝) (Figure 1-5). To preserve its power, the Qing Dynasty suppressed all martial training in China. The Shaolin Temple was completely destroyed at this time.

The early years of the Qing Dynasty saw a mixture of Manchurian and Chinese weapons. In the 1700's, however, the popularity of martial weapons for close-contact fighting started to fade in favor of firearms.

During the Qing Dynasty, there were three places which were famous for their weapons. The first two areas, Long Quan (龍泉) and Wu Kang (武康), are in

Zhejiang Province (浙江省) in eastern China. The third area, Qin Yang (沁陽), is in Henan Province (河南省), site of the Shaolin Temples. Long Quan, although encompassing very little area, attracted great sword makers because of its water. No one knows what qualities the water possesses, but great arms have been forged in Long Chuan for many centuries.

In 1911, Sun, Yat-Sen (孫中山) lead a revolution of the Han people, took power and founded the Republic of China.

The evolution in Chinese weapons, from stones picked from the river to intricately carved swords made of metal alloys to guns, took nearly 5,000 years. Only recently have martial artists sought to resurrect the art of ancient Chinese weapons. Now, martial artists appreciate the weapon as an art form or exercise aid rather than as a necessary tool for combat.

References

1. 槍爲長兵之王，劍爲短兵之首。

2. 百日拳，千日槍，萬日劍。

3. 劍柔，以技見長。刀剛，以力見勝。劍輕手，刀黑走。

4. 刀猛贏之以力，劍軟勝之以技。

5. 刀如猛虎，劍似飛鳳，槍比游龍。

CHAPTER 2

Long Weapons
長兵器

2-1. INTRODUCTION

This chapter includes discussions of both long weapons (five to eight feet in length) and very long weapons (longer than eight feet). Because very long weapons have more specialized uses, only four examples are reviewed, while twenty-five representative long weapons are covered.

These twenty-nine examples are only a small sample of the variety of long weapons. Both the lengths and shapes of these weapons vary considerably. There were no definite patterns or molds from which they were made. The weapon depended on an individual's stature and training. If the martial artist was large and strong, a long, heavy weapon was no problem. But if he did not have great strength, a slightly shorter and lighter weapon served him better.

Generally, big battles featured the long and very long weapons. They were usually used by mounted warriors against other soldiers on horseback. Chariot riders commonly carried long weapons for attacking other chariots. Often, a warrior in a chariot would use a long weapon against an enemy on horseback. Only occasionally did soldiers use long weapons for ground-to-ground fighting.

Very long weapons had a special purpose in addition to those discussed above. They could be used effectively to attack or defend a walled city. Soldiers used extremely long weapons (over 15 feet) to remove defenders from the tops of the walls and gain entry into the city. The defensive forces, of course, utilized similar weapons to prevent entry.

Long weapons provided the martial artist with two major advantages over an enemy carrying a short weapon. First, he had greater killing potential because of the power inherent in the long and heavy weapon. Second, he had a strategic advantage in being able to strike his enemy before the short weapons became effective.

There were disadvantages as well in carrying a long weapon. Endurance became a problem because of the weapon's weight. Also, carrying a long weapon for self-defense was impractical. A short weapon was much easier to transport.

Also, if the enemy was able to get in close, the long weapon lost almost all of its effectiveness.

In spite of all of the disadvantages of long weapons, many famous ancient Chinese generals carried them into battle. Yue Fei (岳飛) (Southern Song Dynasty 1127-1280 A.D., 南宋) and Qi, Ji-Guang (戚繼光) (Ming Dynasty 1368-1644 A.D., 明朝) used spears. Guan Yu (關羽) (Three Kingdoms 220-280 A.D., 三國) chose a long-handled, broad-bladed saber.

In this chapter, ancient Chinese units of length, Chi (尺) (1 Chi=0.3581 meters) are used. No exact conversion to English units is possible because the Chi changed from dynasty to dynasty. Generally speaking, one Chi is slightly less than one foot.

The reader must understand that no definite length or weight exists for any group of weapons. Individual weapons varied among martial artists depending on their physical stature. Measurements given in this book should serve as a rough estimate or average for a group of weapons.

2-2. VERY LONG WEAPONS

Very long weapons are the longest range contact fighting weapons (projectile and thrown weapons, of course, have greater range, but are not for contact fighting). Generally, only the largest and most powerful warriors carried very long weapons.

Such armament was used mainly for horse-to-horse fighting with one notable exception: they were also used by the flag bearers. In a large battle, the major generals or commanding officers were flanked by flags representing the army. The flags, very long weapons in themselves, were carried by the strongest and best-trained men. For protection at short distance, the flag bearers were usually surrounded by soldiers.

Eighteen-Chi Tapered Rod (Shuo, 槊) (Mao-Shuo, 矛槊). In ancient times, weapons such as the long lance, spear or rod, which were especially heavy, resilient and long were called Shuo. The document, *Understanding Correct Words* (正字通) states that the "lance which is as long as eighteen Chi is called Shuo."[1] At the end of the lance or rod, different shapes (e.g., tapered) or specially designed metals were attached to increase the injury potential of the weapon. To increase its strength and resilience, the rod was commonly immersed in tung oil (桐油) (i.e., wood-oil obtained from the seeds of paulownia).

The Shuo was most often used by warriors on horseback against enemies either on horses or in chariots (Figure 2-1). The Shuo was also effective when used by a foot-soldier against a mounted opponent. The great length of this weapon made it ideal for defending or attacking walled cities. During the Liang Jian Wen era (550-551 A.D., 梁簡文帝), general Xiou Gang (蕭綱) wrote a book about the Shuo techniques used in horse back fighting.[2]

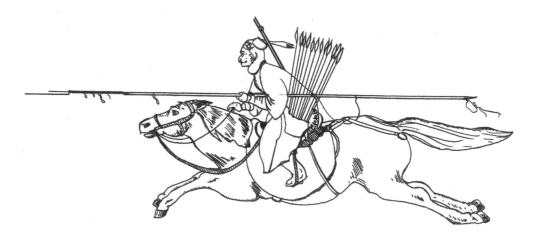

Figure 2-1

The Shuo was used not only for stabbing the enemy, but also for attacking his horse's legs. The resilience of the Shuo was put to use by shaking the thick end and rebounding the tapered end to knock the rider off his horse. However, the Shuo became very awkward at close range.

Examples of the Shuo are first found in the Spring and Autumn Period and the Warring States Period (722-222 B.C., 春秋戰國). It later evolved into the spear during the Han Dynasty(206 B.C.-220 A.D., 漢朝).

Lance or Long Spear (Mao, 矛). The Mao was a straight tapered long rod. In ancient times, a sharpened stone or animal bone was tightened at the end of the rod to increase killing potential. Later, when brass was discovered in beginning in the Shang Dynasty (1751-1111 B.C., 商朝), a brazen point was attached to the end of the lance or spear . This was called the "Brass Lance" (Tong Mao, 銅矛). Often, both sides were tightly fitted with brass to become a "Double Head Mao" (Shuang Tou Mao, 雙頭矛). In ancient times, the length of the metal at the end of the lance was about 25 cm, while the length of the rod varied. For example, the length for the Mao used for chariots was about 7.5 meters; this was called the "Barbarian Mao" (Yi Mao, 夷矛) or "Two Mao" (Er Mao, 二矛). Those used for ground battle were about 6.5 meters, and those used for the horse back battle were about 6 meters. These were commonly called "Eighteen-Chi Snake Lance" (Zhang Ba She Mao, 丈八蛇矛).

The Mao was used not only for stabbing the enemy, but also for attacking his horse's legs. The resiliency of the Mao was put to use by shaking the thick end and rebounding the tapered end to knock the rider off his horse. The Mao was commonly used in chariot fighting, ground battle, and horse back fighting. The Mao became very awkward at close range.

The Mao was created during the Shang Dynasty (1751-1111 B.C., 商朝), and later, in the Jin (265-420 A.D., 晉), Sui (581-618 A.D., 隋), and Tang Dynasties (618-907 A.D., 唐), it was called the Shuo. It is therefore difficult to distinguish the differences between the Mao and the Shuo. That is why these weapons were commonly called Mao-Shuo (矛槊).

Twelve-Chi or Thirteen-Chi Rod (Shu, 殳 or Zhang-Er, 丈二) (Figure 2-2). The Shu was also called "Chu" (杵), "Zhang" (杖), or "Bang," (棒) and was usually made of bamboo or a solid piece of strong wood. Normally, the Shu was twelve to thirteen Chi long. During the Chinese Spring and Autumn period (722-484 B.C., 春秋), and the Warring States period (403-222 B.C., 戰國), the material was gradually changed into metal. It is recorded in the ancient book, *Biographies* (傳) that: "Shu's length is Zhang-Er (twelve Chi) and no sharpened edge."[3]

The Shu was originally used to strike the enemy in a chariot, on horse back, or for ground battle. Later, it was generally used as a weapon to open the path for kings or emperors.[4]

Techniques for the Shu are similar to those of the Shuo, but because it was much lighter, it was most commonly used by weaker soldiers. Also, because of its reduced length and weight, the Shu could be maneuvered with greater speed and flexibility than the Shuo. The general technique for the Shu was the strike. However, if one end of the rod was tapered, it could also be used for stabbing.

During the Xia (2205-1766 B.C., 夏), Shang (1766-1122 B.C., 商), and Zhou (1122-249 B.C., 周) Dynasties, the Shu was classified as one of the five main army weapons.

Nine-Chi Tapered Rod (Jiu-Chi, 九尺) (Figure 2-2). The Jiu-Chi is a nine-Chi tapered rod. The Jiu-Chi was commonly used to strike the enemy in a chariot, on horse back, or for ground battle. Later, it was generally used as a weapon to open a path for kings or emperors. Jiu-Chi was a long weapon commonly used in Southern Chinese martial styles.

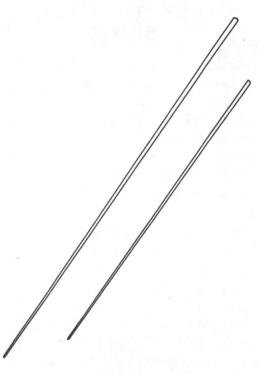

Figure 2-2

Techniques of the Jiu-Chi are similar to those of the Shu, but because it was much lighter, it was more commonly used by a weaker soldier. Also, because of its reduced length and weight, the Jiu-Chi could be maneuvered with greater speed and flexibility than the Shu. The Jiu-Chi was probably created during the same period as the Shu.

2-3. LONG WEAPONS

Long weapons differ from very long weapons by having a greater number of uses. They can be utilized at shorter distances and are especially useful in ground fighting. The shorter length of long weapons allows for various techniques not possible with very long weapons. Also, more long weapons exist than very long weapons. In this section, we will first introduce

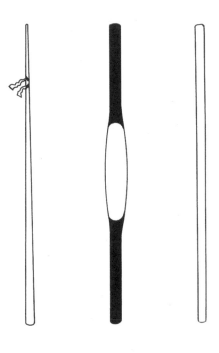

Figure 2-3

the single long weapons and then follow with double long weapons.

Single Long Weapons 單長兵

Rod or Club (Gun, 棍) (Tiao-Zi, 條子) (Figure 2-3). The Gun, or Tiao-Zi in the West and North of China, was generally made of hard wood (e.g., birch or oak). The Gun was often immersed in wood oil to increase its strength and resilience. Occasionally, long rods were made of brass or iron, and were either solid or hollow metal. The former made a heavy and powerful weapon, whereas the latter was designed for lightness and speed. Both types had the distinct advantage of being invulnerable to bladed weapons. The circumference of the long rod was such that the thumb and first finger of its carrier just touched around it. The length of the Gun differed from the North of China to the South. A Northern martial artist carried a long rod that reached the base of his wrist when his arm was extended over his head. The Southern fighter's long rod reached only to his eyebrows. This is why it is called "Equal Eyebrows Rod" (Qi Mei Gun, 齊眉棍).

There are three popular kinds of long rods. The first and most common kind consists of a straight piece of rod. The second kind, called "Water-Fire Rod" (Shui

Huo Gun, 水火棍) has metal caps covering both ends of the rod, but neither end is sharp. The third rod, called "Rod Spear" (Gun Qiang, 棍槍) has one tapered end that can be used for piercing.

The long rod dates from at least the period of Huang Di and probably earlier. It is one of the most convenient and easily utilized weapons. Long pieces of wood can be found anywhere, both on the road and at home.

The most common techniques for Gun are brushing, sweeping, striking and thrusting upwards through the opponent's crotch. Sliding the rod through one hand to utilize either end brings the long rod alive.

Spear (Qiang, 槍**).** The Qiang evolved very early in Chinese history. The Qiang was originally made by tapering the end of a piece of bamboo (Zhu Qiang, 竹槍) (Figure 2-4) or rod (Gun Qiang, 棍槍). The length of the spear varied, depending on the individual's height and purpose. The weapon was later modified by adding a tapered metal head that was sharp on both edges. This kind of spear was also used as a thrown weapon, and was called "Throwing Spear" (Biao Qiang, 標槍) (Figure 2-4). Moreover, horsetail tassels were added to serve two functions. First, they distracted the enemy. Second, and more importantly, they stopped the flow of blood from the blade to the handle after killing the enemy. Therefore, it was called the "blood stopper" (Xue Dang, 血擋) (Figure 2-5). This was crucial because the stickiness of blood on the handle would affect sliding techniques and would render other techniques more dangerous to perform.

In the Southern Song Dynasty(1127-1280 A.D.), it was said that General Yue Fei (岳飛) made a third addition to

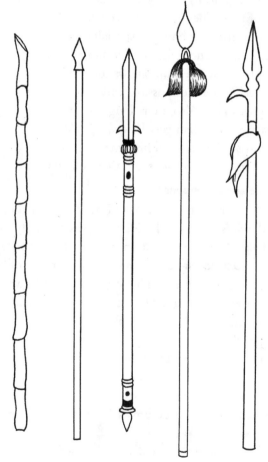

Figure 2-4   Figure 2-5   Figure 2-6

the spear. To the metal end of the spear, he added a hook which was sharp on both edges and could be used for cutting off the legs of horses. This hooking weapon was later called "Hook-Scythe-Spear" (Gou Lian Qiang, 鉤鐮槍) (Figure 2-6) during the Qing Dynasty (1644-1911 A.D., 清朝). There were many designs of the spears or hook spears, depending on the dynasties (Figures 2-7 to 2-9). One of the modifications to the spear was a sharp metal taper on both ends, used to increase the weapon's killing potential. This double spear was called Shuang Tou Qiang (雙頭槍) (Figure 2-10).

The spear body was usually made of "white wax wood" (Bai La Gan, 白臘桿), which only grows in Northern China. Rattan was also utilized, especially in

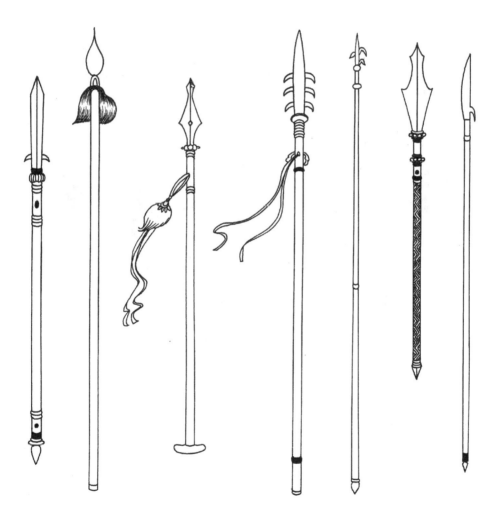

Figure 2-7

Southern China. Both materials are extremely flexible and tough. Often, the wood was soaked in oil for several months to increase its resilience and strength.

The spear was used in battles where both soldiers were mounted, both were on the ground, only one was mounted, or both were in chariots. The spear is called "king of the long weapons" (長兵之王) because its techniques and applications are superior to those of other weapons. It is light and therefore can be used with quickness and agility like a dragon's tail. The main attack technique is stabbing (stinging). When used defensively, the spear can be "wrapped" around an enemy's weapon, forcing it from his grasp. The major disadvantage of the spear is that it cannot block heavy weapons such as a large saber or halberd very well. It is also extremely difficult to master the use of the spear.

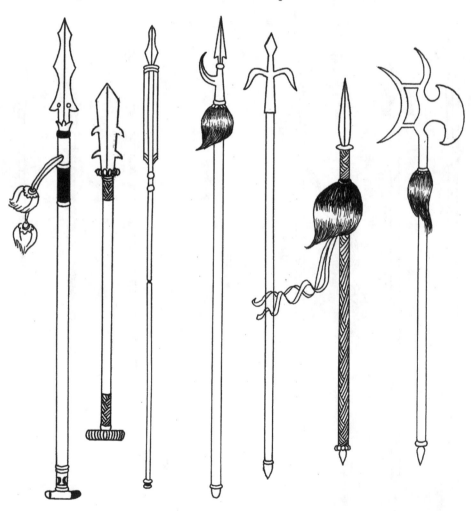

Figure 2-8

According to Chinese weapons history, the Qiang was derived from the Mao (i.e., lance), which was longer and heavier. The Mao was popularly used before the Qin Dynasty (255-206 B.C., 秦朝), and was gradually modified into the long spear. A typical example of the spear at this time was a design mixture of the Mao and the Qiang, called the Mao-Qiang (矛槍) (Figure 2-11). The techniques used were a mixture of both weapons.

It was not until the Jin Dynasty (265-420 A.D., 晉朝) that the spear became shorter and lighter. The apex in the development of the spear probably came in the Southern Song Dynasty (1127-1180 A.D., 宋朝), when General Yue Fei (岳飛) added a sharp, nasty hook near the end. Another general, Qi,

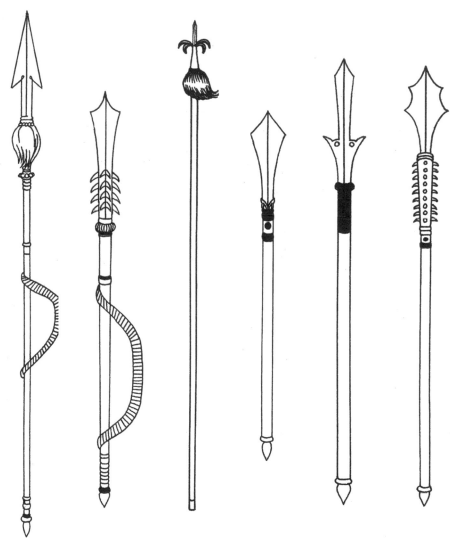

Figure 2-9

Ji-Guang (戚繼光) in the Ming Dynasty (1386-1644 A.D., 明朝) was also a famous spear user.

Long Staff (Chang Bang, 長棒). This weapon is similar to the long rod, but has a very heavy metal addition on one end. This metal sleeve may be serrated, such as in the "Wolf's Teeth Staff" (Lang Ya Bang, 狼牙棒), the "Bone Flower" (Gu Duo, 骨朵), the "Upright Melon" (Li Gua, 立瓜), and the "Lying Melon" (Wo Gua, 臥瓜) (Figure 2-12). Often the opposite or light end of the staff was capped with a small piece of metal.

The Bang can be used either for horseback or ground fighting. The long staff developed with the long rod, but because of its greater weight, it required a stronger person. The techniques of the long staff are also reduced, because it cannot be used equally well on either side. Its use is limited to striking and sweeping. Although its techniques are not as involved as the long rod, the long staff has greater killing potential because of its weight. In addition, the serrations, or "wolf's teeth," tended to intimidate the enemy, making him easier prey. The long staff might have been developed during the same period as the Gun (rod).

Long-Handled Saber (Da Dao, 大刀). There are many different designs for the long-handled saber, which varied during different periods of Chinese history. The key to the long-handled broadsword was its sharp and extremely heavy metal head (approximately 40 pounds), which was common to all long-handled sabers.

The most popular long-handled saber was called "Guan's Long-Handled Saber"

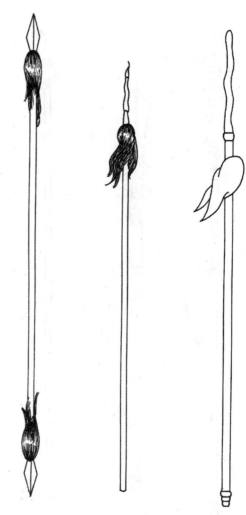

Figure 2-10

Figure 2-11

(Guan Dao, 關刀). Guan Dao began in the Chinese Three Kingdoms Period (221-280 A.D.) and was used by Guan Yu (or Guan, Yun-Chang) (關羽；關雲長). His Long-Handled Saber was called "Green-Dragon Scything-Moon Saber," (Qing Long Yan Yue Dao, 青龍偃月刀) or simply "Green Dragon Saber" (Qing Long Dao, 青龍刀) (Figure 2-13). The Guan Dao was very heavy, and it required great strength to handle it in battle. It is thought that this weapon was about eight Chi long, and weighed nearly ninety pounds. Therefore it was not practical for most people, who did not possess the great strength of General Guan. The Guan Dao has been commonly used for training purposes, to build strength and endurance.[5] Generally, the saber of the Guan Dao had a notch or hook in it for catching and

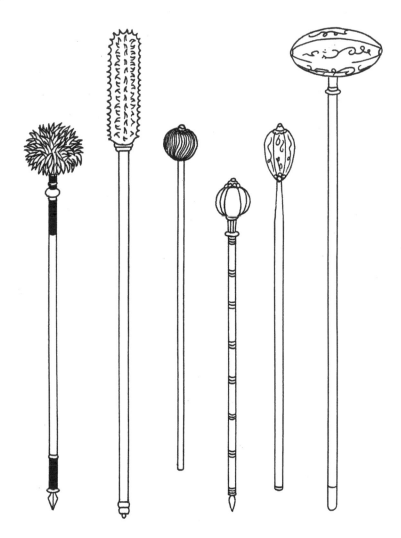

Figure 2-12

parrying an enemy's weapon. The tassel on the saber was only for distraction. The hand protection (Hu Shou, 護手), at the base of the blade, was used to stop blood from flowing down to the handle, and also to prevent the enemy's weapon from sliding on to the user's hand. The handle was made of either metal or a hardwood that had been soaked in oil. A small piece of metal capped the handle's end.

One kind of long-handled saber was named "Dashing Saber" (Pu Dao, 撲刀) by northern Chinese martial artists, or "Kick Saber" (Ti Dao, 踢刀) and "Cai Yang's Saber" (Cai Yang Dao, 蔡陽刀) by southern Chinese martial artists (Figure 2-14). This kind of saber did not have a notch or hook on the saber blade. Sometimes it had rings on the back of the blade which would rattle and make noise to scare and distract the enemy. Pu Dao, which had a shorter rod and longer saber

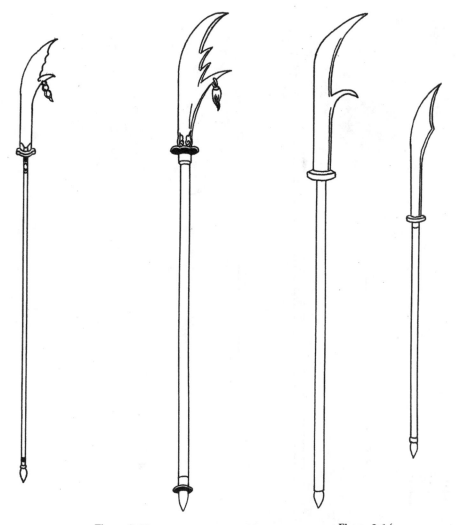

Figure 2-13   Figure 2-14

blade, was called "Yue Fei's Long-Handled Saber (Yue Fei Da Dao, 岳飛大刀). It is said that this kind of saber was created by Marshal Yue Fei, who used it to attack the legs of the enemy's horses.

There are also many other long-handled sabers, designed for different purposes and created in different historical periods. These long-handled sabers are: "Hook Sickle Saber" (Gou Lian Dao, 鉤鐮刀), "Elephant Nose Long-Handled Saber" (Xiang-Bi Da Dao, 象鼻大刀), "Eyebrow Tip Saber" (Mei Jian Dao, 眉尖刀), "Brush Saber" (Bi Dao, 筆刀), and "Slide Saber" or "Thin Saber" (Pian Dao, 片刀) (Figure 2-15). All of these long-handled sabers are sharp only on one side of the blade.

There are also some other designs which are considered to be long-handled sabers, in which both sides of the metal head are sharp and on which the tips

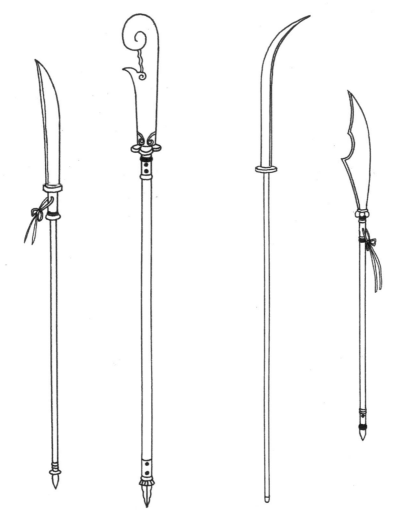

Figure 2-15

have been pointed for piercing. Some of the examples are: "Wind Mouth Saber" (Feng Zui Dao, 風嘴刀), "Erlang's Saber" (Erlang's Dao, 二郎刀), "He-wolf Ear Saber" (Huan Er Dao, 獾耳刀), and "Wagging Saber" (Diao Dao, 掉刀) (Figure 2-16).

Long-handled sabers were generally used for horse-to-horse fighting. However, some of the lighter ones were also commonly used for ground-versus-horseback (to chop the horse's legs) and ground-to-ground fighting.

Shovel or Spade (Chan, 鏟). The general structure of the shovel is a flat metal head on the end of a metal rod, or a rod made from strong wood. A small metal piece covers the opposite end of the rod (Figure 2-17). Three different shovels or

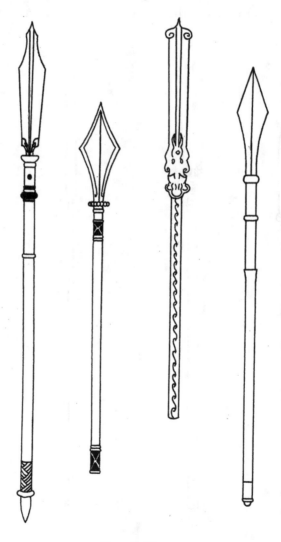

Figure 2-16

spades are commonly known. The "Crescent Moon Shovel" (Yue Ya Chan, 月牙鏟) has a moon-shaped head, sometimes adorned with metal rings (Figure 2-18). The "Convenient Shovel" (Fang Bian Chan, 方便鏟) was mainly constructed from a piece of flat metal sharpened at the edge. Often, the other end was given a convex, moon-shaped blade of metal, which was adorned with rings (Figure 2-19). The "Golden Coin Shovel" (Jin Qian Chan, 金錢鏟) has a coin-shaped metal head (Figure 2-20). There are also other shapes for the shovel, the design of which depended on their purposes during different periods of Chinese history. For example, "Heaven Tangled Shovel" (Tian Peng Chan, 天蓬鏟) was designed during the Ming Dynasty (1638-1644 A.D., 明朝) for use by foot soldiers (Figure 2-21).[6] Another kind of shovel, called "Lotus Flower Shovel" (Lian Hua Chan, 蓮花鏟), had one end crowned with a moon-shaped metal blade, while the other

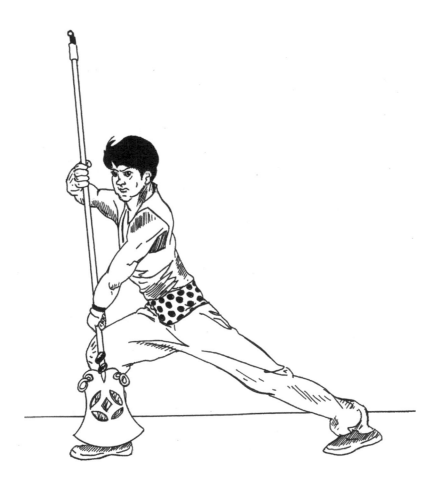

Figure 2-17

end had a lotus flower-shaped metal cap, which was used to balance the weight on both ends (Figure 2-22).

The use of the shovel began in the stone age. The blade of the shovel in this time was comprised of a sharp edge of stone. Later, when brass became available during the Shang Dynasty (1766-1122 B.C., 商朝), the stone blade was replaced with brass. It was not until China's late Warring States Period (403-222 B.C., 戰國) that iron was used, and the weapon became even sharper. The "Crescent Moon Shovel" was created during the Ming Dynasty (1638-1644 A.D., 明朝), and since then has become a popular martial arts long weapon. The "Golden Bell Shovel"

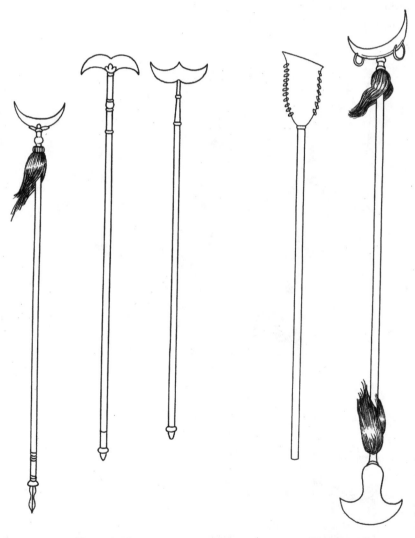

Figure 2-18   Figure 2-19

(Jin Zhong Chan, 金鐘鏟) is a very ancient weapon, made with a stone head. Legend says that Emperor Yu, of the Xia Dynasty (2205-1766 B.C.) (夏禹), was a master of the golden bell shovel.

After Buddhism migrated to China from India during the Han Dynasty (206 B.C.-25 A.D., 漢朝), the shovel became the weapon of priests. They used it to dig holes to bury the dead following the wars and famines that ravaged ancient China. They also used the shovels as defense weapons when they traveled. In fact, the crescent moon shovel remained exclusively a monk's weapon until the end of the Qing Dynasty (1644-1911 A.D., 清朝).

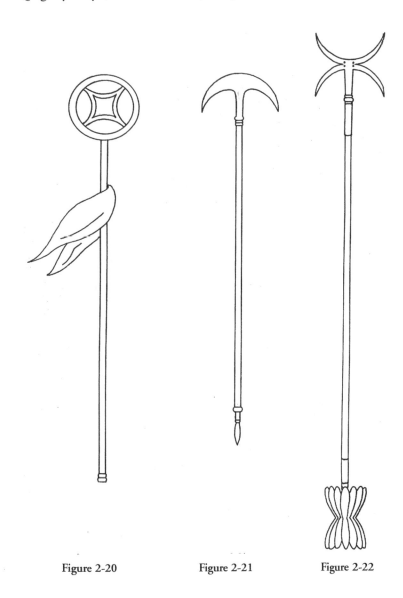

Figure 2-20   Figure 2-21   Figure 2-22

The head of a shovel can be used to attack the opponent's head, or to chop the foot. The crescent moon shape of the blade can be used to hook the enemy's weapon. When its user's back was against the wind, the shovel could also be used to scoop up dirt and throw it into the opponent's eyes, blinding him for the fight.[6]

Fork (Cha, 叉). The fork can be divided into two types, one with three tines, commonly called "Trident or Three-Tined Fork" (San Cha or San Gu Cha, 三叉、三股叉) (Figure 2-23), and the other with two tines, called different names depending on the purpose. Because the trident became a common hunting weapon which was often thrown, it is also called "Flying Fork" (Fei Cha or Bian Cha, 飛叉、標叉). Different names were sometimes given, according to different designs

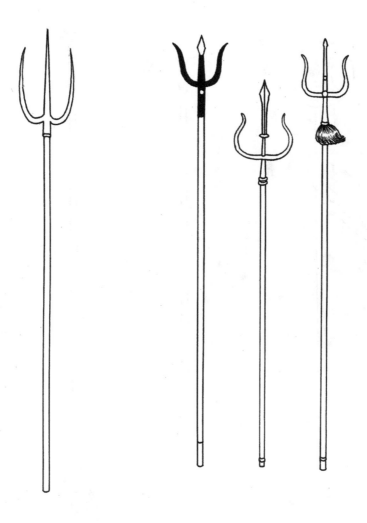

Figure 2-23   Figure 2-24

or purposes, such as "Horse Fork" (Ma Cha, 馬叉), "Steel Fork" (Gang Cha, 鋼叉), and "Scholar Fork" (Wen Cha, 文叉) (Figure 2-24). The only known two-tined forks are "Fire Fork" (Huo Cha, 火叉) and "Fork Staff" (Cha Gan, 叉竿) (Figure 2-25).

In this design, a three-tined or two-tined metal head was attached to a wooden rod. Occasionally a metal staff was used. The weapon was slightly longer than the user's body. The trident differed in Northern and Southern China. In the North, the tines were flat with sharp edges and points in contrast to the tapered tines of the South.

The trident was mainly a hunting tool, and not a favorite battle weapon. The trident was thought to scare off evil spirits, so many families and temples kept them near. The trident was also commonly used as a martial artist's performance weapon (Figure 2-26).

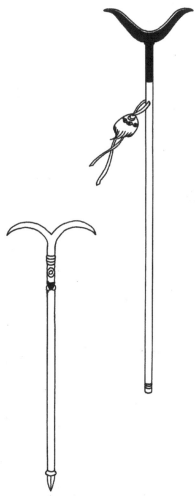

As a fighting weapon, the trident was used to block and lock the enemy's weapon. Offensively, it was used either to stab or sweep. In hunting tigers, the hunter would hold the trident tilted upward at a 45 degrees angle, with the butt anchored into something solid. Sometimes the hunter would leave the trident lying flat on the ground, and raise it up only as the tiger pounced. As the tiger jumped in to attack, it would impale itself on the weapon.

Rake (Ba and Tang,
鈀、耙、扒、杷、鑡). There are many different Chinese characters which represent the rake (Ba). All of these characters are pronounced the same way. This may be because most Chinese were illiterate in ancient times, which lead to the different ways for expressing the rake in writing.

The rake resembles a modern, Western rake. It was a wooden rod with wooden or metal "fingers" at the head. As with other weapons, different designs of the rake were generated

Figure 2-25

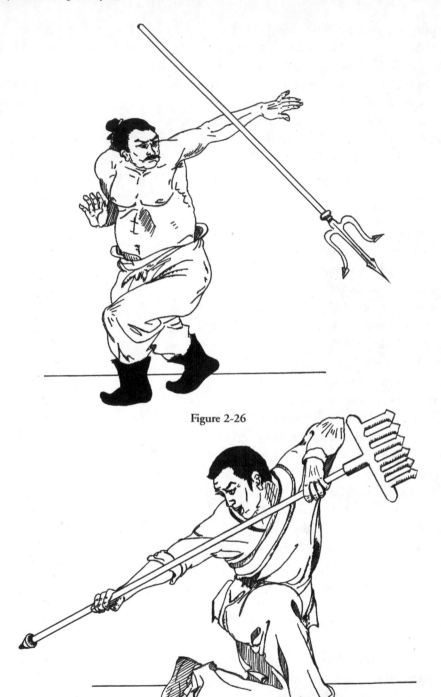

Figure 2-26

Figure 2-27

depending on the time and the area. The rake was originally designed for agricultural purposes. Farmers learned to utilize it to defend against bandits and protect their property. Farmers often trained to use all of their farming tools as weapons (Figure 2-27). The most ancient rakes were made of wood (Figure 2-28). Later, the head was fitted with sharp, pointed metal fingers (Figure 2-29). The rake dates from before Shen Nong (2737 B.C., 神農) when it was used as a farming tool.

Another kind of weapon, called the "Tang" (鏜) was similar to the "Ba." However, the metal part was constructed from a crescent moon-shaped piece of metal, very similar to the Shovel discussed earlier (Figure 2-30). When the designs

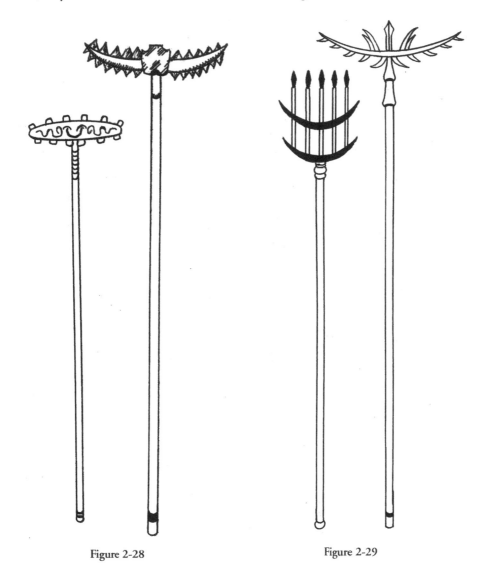

Figure 2-28   Figure 2-29

of the rake and Tang were mixed, it was called "Tang-Ba" (Figure 2-31). The Tang or Ba is often confused with the "Fork" (Cha, 叉). Sometimes, the Fork is called "Da Ba" (Large Rake, 大鈀) in northern China.

L-Shaped Lance (Flat-Head Halberd) (Ge, 戈). At first the Ge was built by using an animal horn or a sharp stone connected to the end of a long rod. It was used for hunting and fighting, and was called "Stone Ge" (Shi Ge, 石戈). Later, the stone was replaced with brass. The edge of the metal head was then sharpened for hooking and stabbing (Figure 2-32). The rod attached to the metal head could be long or short. When it was short, it was called "Short Ge" (Duan Ge, 短戈) and was classified as a short weapon. When it was long, it was called "Long Ge" (Chang Ge, 長戈) and was classified as a long weapon.

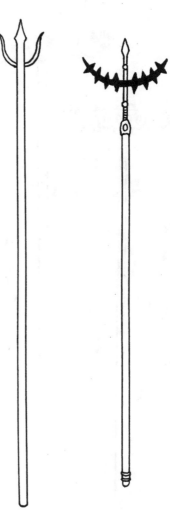

The Ge was the main hunting weapon in ancient times. In battle, the long Ge was commonly used in horseback-to-horseback or chariot fighting, while the short Ge was used in ground-to-ground battle.

The main use of the Ge is to hook, to peck, and to stab the opponent. The Ge was one of the major heavy weapons before the Spring and Autumn Period and Warring States Period (722-222 B.C., 春秋戰國). After the Qin Dynasty (255-206 B.C., 秦朝), the Ge gradually disappeared from the battlefield.

Halberd (Ji, 戟). In structure, the Ji can be considered to be a mixture of the Mao and the Ge. There are many kinds of halberds. The two which are most alike and well known are the "Sky Halberd" (Fang Tian Hua Ji, 方天畫戟) and the "Horse Halberd" (Ma Ji, 馬戟) (Figure 2-33). With the Sky Halberd, there are two crescent moon shapes on the sides, with a sharp spear head pointing forward, while on the Horse Halberd there is only one crescent moon shape on the side. The rod is generally made of hard wood or metal.

Figure 2-30   **Figure 2-31**

Horsetail tassels are used both to distract the enemy and to prevent blood from flowing down the shaft.

The primary purpose of the halberd was in horseback-to-horseback fighting though it may have also been used in horseback-to-ground and ground-to-ground battles. Stabbing and hooking were the primary techniques executed with the halberd. Thrusting upwards, sweeping, sliding and cutting were also performed.

The first brass Ji was created at the beginning of the Shang Dynasty (1766-1122 B.C., 商朝). In the Zhou Dynasty, the main design of the Ji was a mixture of the Mao and the Ge. The material of the Ji's head was brass. In the Spring and Autumn Period (722-484 B.C., 春秋), the Ji was considered to be a major weapon in big battles. Near the end of the Warring States Period (403-222 B.C., 戰國), brass was replaced by iron to create a stronger weapon. From the Western Han Dynasty (206 B.C.-25 A.D., 西漢) to the Western Jin Dynasty (265-317 A.D., 西晉), the Ji was con-

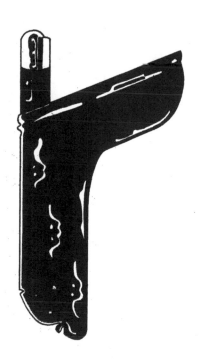

Figure 2-32

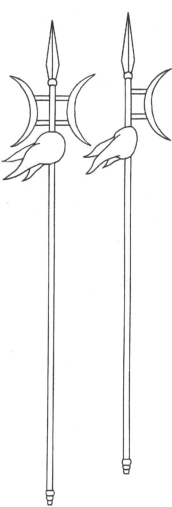

Figure 2-33

39

sidered to be one of the five main battle weapons. Its popularity expanded greatly during the Three Kingdoms era (220-265 A.D., 三國). The famous general, Lu Bu (呂布), during the Three Kingdoms era favored halberds for their great killing potential. After this, the usefulness of the Ji gradually became downgraded. In fact, the Ji in the Tang Dynasty (618-907 A.D., 唐朝) was used only for military decoration and ceremony, such as the "Qi-Ji" (Enveloped-Halberd, 棨戟) and the "Ji-Dao" (Halberd-Saber, 戟刀) (Figure 2-34).

Long-Handled Battle Axe (Yue, 鉞). The Short-Handled Battle Axe was called "Fu" (斧) while the Long-Handled Battle Axe was called "Yue" (鉞). The Yue is therefore commonly called "Da Fu" (Large Axe, 大斧) (Figure 2-35). The axe was

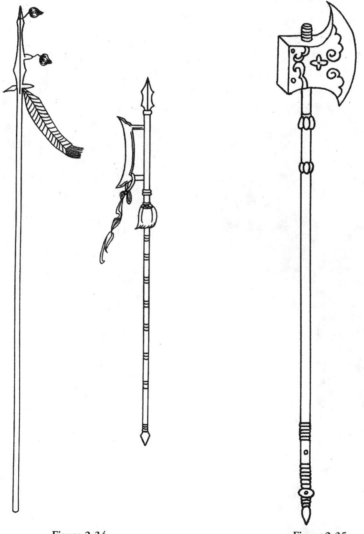

Figure 2-34   Figure 2-35

originally used for chopping wood, and later became a battle weapon. The long-handled axe was used primarily for horseback-to-horseback fighting in large battles, while foot soldiers used shorter versions.

Chopping and stabbing were common techniques of the axe. The disadvantages of the battle axe were that the staff was not flexible, and it was extremely heavy. The axe was created as soon as metal became available in ancient times. It was gradually disregarded, simply because its weight and awkwardness of handling.

Brush, Brush Attacker, Brass Fist (Bi, Bi Zhua, Tong Quan, 筆、筆檛、銅拳). The brush, brush attacker and brass fist each consisted of a long wooden or metal

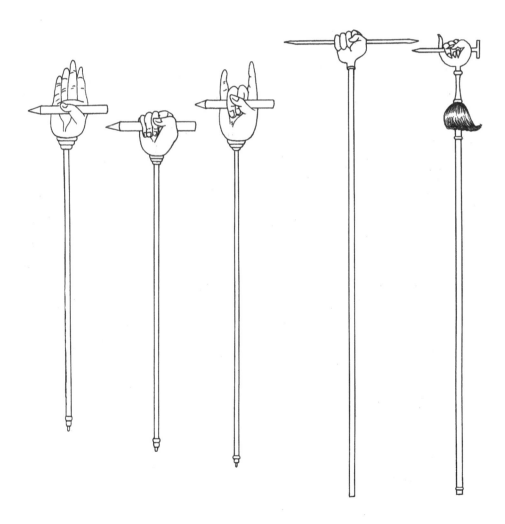

Figure 2-36

staff, with a metal hand-shaped end holding a very sharp metal pen, brush or even a fist (Figure 2-36). Sometimes, only a metal fist was installed. These kinds of weapons were used in horseback-to-horseback fighting. These weapons may have developed during the Chinese Song Dynasty (960-1280 A.D., 宋朝).

Long-Handled Sickle (Da Lian, 大鐮). The Long-Handled Sickle is also commonly called "Large Sickle" (Da Lian, 大鐮). On the side of one end, the hooked sickle was designed both with and without a spear head. Therefore, the techniques of the spear and sickle can be mixed. There are different designs of the long-handled sickle, including the "Fire Sickle" (Huo Lian, 火鐮), the "Large Sickle" (Da Lian, 大鐮), and the "Jade Sickle" (Yu Lian, 玉鐮) (Figure 2-37).

Long-handled sickles were developed when metal became available. Their popularity peaked during the Chinese Song Dynasty (960-1280 A.D., 宋朝), and then gradually disappeared from the battle field.

Long-Handled Claw (Zhua, 抓). The Zhua consists of a metal or wooden rod ending in a metal hand with sharp fingers or claws (Figure 2-38). The Long-Handled Claw was used in big battles in ancient times. The main technique was using the claw to hook or to injure the opponent. The Long-Handled Claw may have been developed during the Chinese Han Dynasty (206 B.C.-220 A.D., 漢朝).

Hoe (Ba Tou, 把頭). Like the modern hoe, the Ba Tou has a flat metal head attached to a wooden handle. The Hoe was a farmer's tool which, when necessary, would be used as a weapon (Figure 2-39). The history of using the hoe as a weapon can be traced back to the emperor Shen Nong (2737 B.C., 神農).

Buddha Hand (Fo Shou, 佛手). The Buddha hand resembles the pen or brush, except that it lacks the sharp

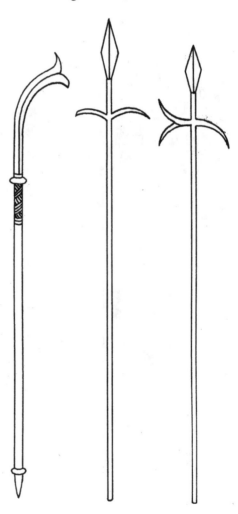

Figure 2-37

point of the pen. The hand is made of metal, and the handle might be metal or wood (Figure 2-40). Like the pen, the Buddha hand was used mainly by priests for non-lethal defense. The Buddha hand originated in the Han Dynasty (206 B.C.-220 A.D., 漢朝).

Other Miscellaneous Long-Handled Weapons.

There are many other different designs for long weapons. However, their developmental history, usage and techniques are unknown to this author. We will list some of these weapons here.[7]

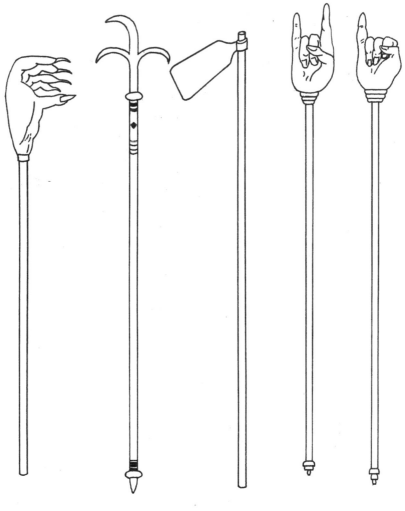

Figure 2-38   Figure 2-39   Figure 2-40

Fire Hook (Huo Gou, 火鉤) (Figure 2-41). Based on the name, we can suppose that this weapon was probably originally used to deal with fire. How it became a weapon is unknown. We only know that this weapon existed during the Chinese Song Dynasty (960-1280 A.D., 宋朝). From its design, we can see that hooking and sliding were probably the main techniques.[8]

Stirring Heaven Killer (Hun Tian Lu, 混天戮) (Figure 2-42). The history of this weapon is unknown. It is only known that this weapon was in existence during the Chinese Ming Dynasty, and was used by the martial artist Li, Cun-Xiao (李存孝).[9] From the design of this weapon, we can see its techniques were probably very similar to those of the Halberd (戟).

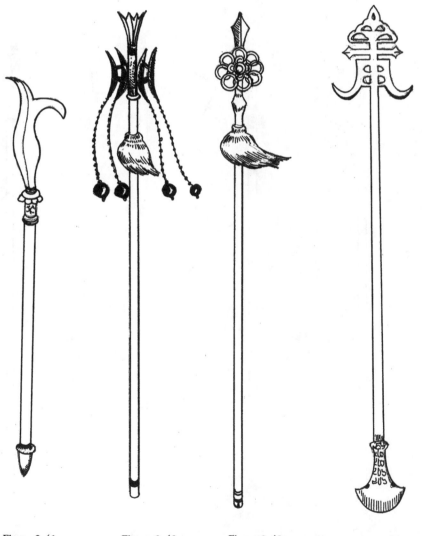

Figure 2-41   Figure 2-42   Figure 2-43   Figure 2-44

Tree Knot (Chun Jie, 枕結) (Figure 2-43). The Chun (枕) is a kind of tree similar to *Ailanthus altissima*. Obviously, this weapon was named for the structure of the knot at its head. This weapon was mentioned in ancient weaponry books. However, no details were given.[10]

Heaven Lotus Wind Tail Tan (Tian He Feng Wei Tan, 天荷風尾鐔) (Figure 2-44). The history of this weapon is unknown. Tan (鐔) is the name of the weapon, but there is no exact translation which can be given. This weapon was constructed out of a shovel (鏟) on one end, and a similar wind-tail hook and sharp-bladed head on the other end. From the design of this weapon, we can see that the main techniques for this weapon were probably mixed with those of the shovel, and also included hooking and stabbing.[7]

Wolf Brush (Lang Xian, 狼筅) (Figure 2-45). The Wolf Brush was created during the Ming Dynasty (1368-1644 A.D., 明朝) and was one of the weapons used to defend against Japanese pirates who constantly harassed China's southeast coast. This weapon was constructed from a spear head, surrounded by branch-like or thorn-like sharp spines which were made from either bamboo or metal. From

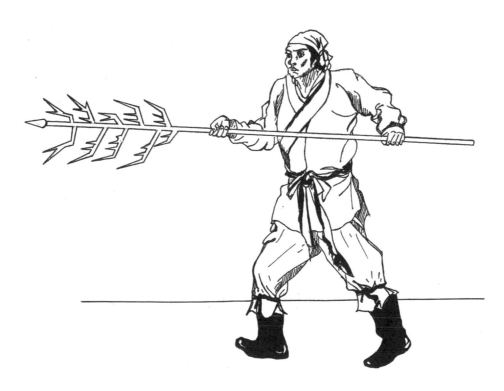

Figure 2-45

the design of this weapon, we can see that it was most likely used to stab or to prevent the enemy's advance.[11]

Lamp Staff (Deng Zhang, 鐙仗 **) (Figure 2-46).** The Lamp Staff was used as a weapon by infantry soldiers to clear a path for the king or emperor.[12] It is not a battle weapon, and is designed to have no sharp edges.

Long-Handled Pincers (Chang Jiao Qian, 長腳鉗 **) (Figure 2-47).** This long weapon looks like a fork (叉). However, according to its name, this weapon was probably used to clamp the opponent's weapon, neck, or limbs. The details of its history and techniques are unknown.[10]

Inviting to Pull Staff (Qing Ren Ba, 請人拔 **) (Figure 2-48).** This weapon is also called "two persons struggling" (Er Ren Duo, 二人奪). The reason for this

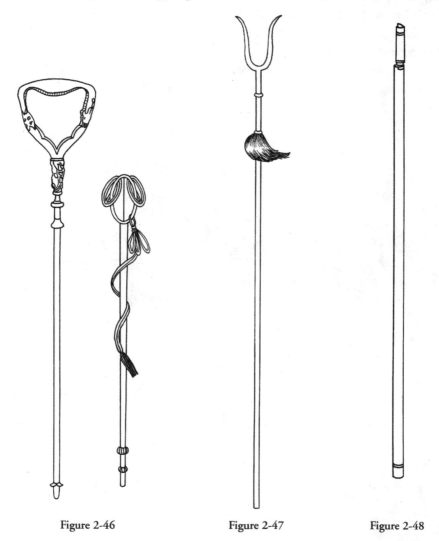

Figure 2-46　　　　　　　　Figure 2-47　　　　　　　　Figure 2-48

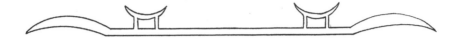

Figure 2-49

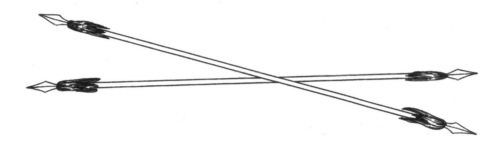

Figure 2-50

name is that there is a sword hidden in the staff. If the opponent grabs the staff and struggles with you, you can pull out the sword and attack him.[10]

Heaven-Earth Sun-Moon Saber (Qian Kun R Yue Dao, 乾坤日月刀). This is a very rare weapon.[7] Its length is about two meters. Both ends have curved, sharp knives. Between the two knives are two handles, which are protected by the two hooked sabers (Figure 2-49). Where this weapon came from is unknown. From the design of the weapon, we can see that it is a ground fighting weapon. The disadvantage of this weapon is that it is hard to carry.

Double Long Weapons 雙長兵

Due to their weight and length, almost all long weapons require handling with both hands. There have therefore never been too many double long weapons. Here, we will introduce the only double long weapon which is known.

Double-Headed Spear (Shuang Tou Qiang, 雙頭槍) (Figure 2-50). Generally speaking, the double-headed spear is shorter than the regular, single-headed spear. Moreover, except for the spear head, most of the spear was made from wood or rattan. This made the spear very light. It was for this reason that some martial artists in the past used the double-headed spear as a one-handed long weapon, allowing two to be used at once, one in each hand.

References

1. 《正字通》說：“矛長丈八謂之槊。”

2. Zhongguo Wushu（〔中國武術實用大全〕，康戈武編著。今日中國出版社。北京。), 1990.

3. 《傳》：“殳長丈二而無刃。”

4. 《詩·衛風·伯氏》：“伯也執殳，為王前驅。”

5. 明茅元儀《武備志》卷一百零三《軍資乘·器械》：“偃月刀以之操習示雄，實不可施于陣也。”

6. 明王圻《三才圖繪·器用》卷八：“形如月牙，內外皆鋒，刃橫長二尺，柄長八九尺，或一丈。兵馬步戰第一利器，直推可以削手，往上推則鏟首，向下推則鏟足，或鉤敗卒之足，或于上風揚塵，妙不勝述。”

7. *Chinese Wushu Great Dictionary*（〔中國武術大辭典〕，人民體育出版社。1990.

8. 宋曾公亮《武經總要》：“火鉤以雙鉤刀為刃。”

9. 明王圻《三才圖繪·器用八卷·兵器類》：“混天戟為李存孝所用

10. 明王圻《三才圖繪·器用八卷·兵器類》。

11. 明戚繼光《紀效新書》卷六《比較武藝賞罰篇》：“凡狼筅，各要利刃在頂，長一尺，四面竹枝，須堅直粗大者。”同書卷十一《狼筅總說篇》：“狼筅之為器也，形體重滯，轉移艱難，非若他枝之出入便捷，似非利器也。殊不知為行伍之藩籬，一軍之門戶。”

12. 宋徐克《高麗圖經》：“鐙仗之設，國王受詔則有之，上為馬鐙其竿丹漆使者前驅千牛衛軍數十八執之，王行則在前，而鐙以涂金為飾，金制悉以鐵為之。”

CHAPTER 3

Short Weapons

短 兵 器

3-1. INTRODUCTION

Short weapons, like their long counterparts, can be divided into two classes based on length. Very short weapons measure less than two Chi (approximately two feet). Often they are no longer than the distance from the hand to the elbow. Short weapons range in length from two to five Chi.

All short weapons possess an inherent advantage over long weapons: they are easy to carry. The same attributes that give short weapons this advantage make them impractical for large battles. They are more effective at short range, and therefore are used more for personal defense than for attack.

It is impossible to discuss all of the short weapons of China. From their birth some 5,000 years ago, short weapons have evolved in such numbers as to make any detailed examination a life's work. This chapter gives only a brief introduction to the more common short weapons. It reviews very short weapons and short weapons.

3-2. VERY SHORT WEAPONS

In this section, we will introduce very short weapons. As mentioned earlier, very short weapons were usually less than two Chi in length. Since they were relatively lighter than longer weapons, very short weapons were also commonly used as throwing weapons. Due to their size, they could be carried easily or hidden somewhere on the body. The disadvantage of very short weapons was that their defensive range was relatively shorter than that of other weapons. In order to increase their defensive capability, very short weapons were commonly used as double weapons. Because of this, we will not divide the very short weapons into "single very short weapons" and "double very short weapons."

Short Sword (Duan Jian, 短劍) (Figure 3-1). The structure of the short sword was the same as that of the regular sword, except that it was shorter and the blade was not as wide. The advantages of the short sword were that it could be hidden and carried easily as a secondary defensive weapon. In addition, if a handkerchief or a piece of cloth was added to the pommel, it could be used as a thrown weapon. When it was used as an thrown weapon, it was called "Flying Sword" (飛劍).

Because it was shorter than the regular sword, the material of the short sword could be a harder steel, and it could therefore be a sharper and stronger weapon. Almost all famously sharp swords are short. Normally, short swords were carried in a pair, and were used in both hands at the same time.

The history of the short sword can be traced back to the very beginning of Chinese weapons smithing. During the Huang Di period (2597-2597 B.C., 黃帝), there already existed short swords made from jade.

Short Saber (Duan Dao, 短刀) (Figure 3-2). Similar to the short sword, the short saber was also only a shorter variation of the regular saber. Again, it could be carried easily and could be hidden on the body, such as in a boot or in the waist area, without the opponent noticing. Moreover, it could be thrown if a piece of cloth was attached to the pommel, which gave it the name "Flying Saber" (Fei Dao, 飛刀). Often short sabers were used in pairs.

The history of the short saber can be traced back to the very beginning of Chinese weapons smithing, during the Huang Di period (2597-2597 B.C., 黃帝).

Iron Ruler (Tie Chi, 鐵尺) (Figure 3-3). The simplest iron ruler was merely a flat metal rod that might or might not be tapered. Some iron rulers had a separate handle. Because the iron ruler was short and easy to carry, it was commonly used by peace officers, in the way a nightstick is used

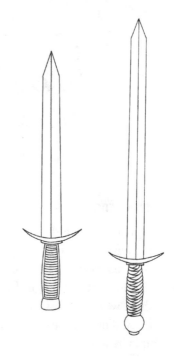

Figure 3-1

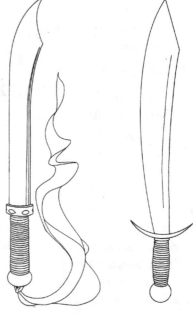

Figure 3-2

by policemen in the West. The iron ruler originated in the Spring and Autumn Period and Warring States Period (722-222 B.C., 春秋戰國).

Scrape Saber (Xiao Dao, 削刀) (**Figure 3-4**). The blade of the scrape saber was metal, and only one edge was sharp. A groove along the blade equalized pressure inside and outside the body, so that the blade could be withdrawn after stabbing. If no groove were present, the vacuum inside the body cavity would hold in the blade.

Like all very short weapons, the scrape saber served as a secondary weapon, used in emergencies, such as the loss of a major weapon. The scrape saber could be hidden by attaching it to the forearm with straps, or it might be hidden in a boot.

The scrape saber, like the dagger, was used for stabbing and cutting. Often, martial artists carried two sabers. The scrape saber could also be used as a throwing weapon. The scrape saber was probably invented during the Spring and Autumn Period and Warring States Period (722-222 B.C.).

Sleeve Sword (Xiou Li Jian, 袖裡劍) (**Figure 3-5**). The sleeve sword was similar to the scrape saber, except that the sleeve sword was straight, and both edges of the blade were sharp. In addition, a spring hidden in the blade could be activated, expanding the weapon to twice its length.

This hidden spring action provided for surprise attack at close range. The sleeve sword was so named because the weapon was traditionally hidden in the sleeves.

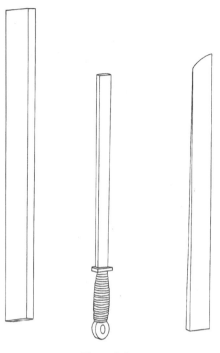

Figure 3-3

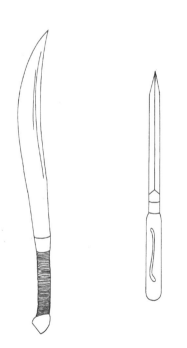

Figure 3-4   Figure 3-5

Techniques for the sleeve sword resembled those of the short sword, except for the surprise lengthening of the blade. When the sleeve sword was extended, normal sword techniques would then be applied. The sleeve sword originated during the Spring and Autumn Period (722-484 B.C.).

Short Trident (Duan Cha, 短又) **(Figure 3-6).** The short trident was a variation of the regular, long trident. The short trident differed in that it was lighter and could be carried easily. The short trident was often used in a pair. The short trident could also be used as a thrown weapon.

As with the long trident, the short trident was originally used as a hunting tool, and only later was it used as a defensive weapon against bandits. As with the long trident, the short trident originated once metal had become available.

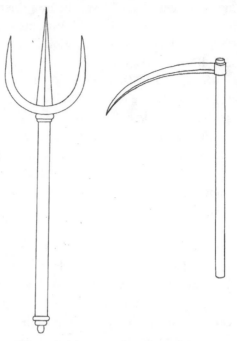

Figure 3-6

Figure 3-7

Sickle (Lian, 鐮) (Figure 3-7). Like a modern sickle, the Lian had a curved, metal head, sharp on one edge and attached to a wooden handle. The sickle was a farmers' tool, originally designed for cutting hay, cane or straw; it later came to be used as a weapon. In ancient China, bandits often gathered by the thousands to rob villages. In order to protect both property and lives, martial arts training was common. Farming and hunting tools were naturally modified into fighting weapons.

Hooking, cutting and striking were common techniques for the sickle. Rarely, the sickle was held by a chain attached to the handle and thrown.

The Lian dates from before Shen Nong (2737 B.C., 神農). Originally, only a sharpened stone blade was attached to a rod. Later, when metal became available, the stone blade was replaced with metal.

Brush Rake Trident (Bi Jia Cha, 筆架又) (Figure 3-8). The words "brush rake" are because this weapon was like

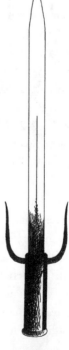

Figure 3-8

the brush rake, and "trident" was because it resembled a trident. This kind of trident differed in that the middle, long piece was like a sword, while the side pieces were like a fork. The length of this trident was about 1.5 Chi. It was commonly used by southern martial styles such as White Crane or Tiger Claw styles. This kind of weapon was commonly used in China's Fujian Province (福建省).

Flute (Xiao or Di, 簫、笛) (Figure 3-9). The flute, a musical instrument adapted for martial arts, was originally made of bamboo. Flutes were later made of iron, steel, brass, or other metals and alloys. A short dagger or sword would often be hidden inside.

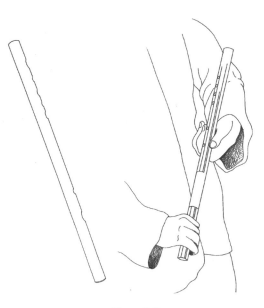

Figure 3-9

The flute alone had little killing potential. Surprise attack came from a hidden dagger or spring loaded darts hidden within. The flute, used as purely a defensive weapon, could be utilized for blocking enemy weapons, while the hidden dagger could be used for stabbing.

The flute dates from very ancient Chinese history. Scholars and martial artists enjoyed music and often carried flutes. It easily evolved into a defensive weapon.

Cymbals (Ba or Nao, 鈸、鐃) (Figure 3-10). The cymbal was a musical instrument. However, it could also be used as a weapon because of its sharp edges. Cymbals were held by a small knob and a cloth ring. Usually, cymbals were made of brass.

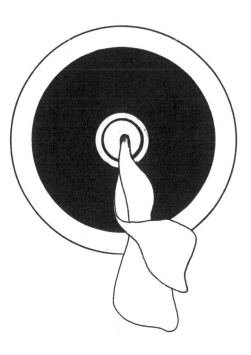

Figure 3-10

The cymbals, like many other ordinary appliances, became serious weapons in the hands of a martial artist. Very few people were familiar with the cymbals as weapons; therefore, they were not easily defended against.

Cymbals could be used to slap, chop, slash or cut. In addition, they could be thrown. Throwing cymbals, called "Nao," were generally smaller. They were called "Flying Nao" (Fei Nao, 飛鐃), and often had serrated edges. When thrown, the cymbal acted like the flying discs used today for recreation. The techniques for throwing were also like those for such flying discs. Cymbals had an advantage over most other weapons in that they constantly emitted a loud and harsh noise, distracting and confusing an opponent.

Cymbals imported from Tibet have been used as musical instruments for thousands of years. Their transition from instruments to weapons occurred during the Tang Dynasty (618-907 A.D., 唐朝).

Fan (Shan, 扇) (Figure 3-11). Fans used by martial artists were made of wood (bamboo and other kinds), or more commonly, metal. The outer edge was extremely sharp, and often spring-loaded darts were hidden in the ribs.

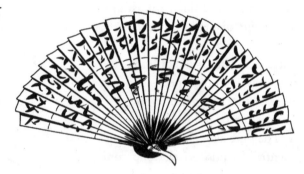

Figure 3-11

Fans were perhaps the most easily hidden weapons, because they could be kept in plain sight. A martial artist with a fan in his hand could at one moment be the elegant scholar, and in the next, a deadly fighter.

Fans, with their razor-sharp edges, could be used to cut, strike or slide. Spring-loaded darts were utilized for surprise attacks. In China, fans are both practical and beautiful, and their use began very early in Chinese history.

Dagger (Bi Shou, 匕首) (Figure 3-12). The dagger has had a long history, even before the Chinese Shang Dynasty (1766-1122 B.C., 商). At that time, it was made from stone or jade. After the Shang Dynasty, these materials were replaced with brass or iron. The dagger has been one of the most popular hidden weapons. It could be carried easily at the waist or in the boot. When necessary, it could be an effective and fast acting weapon for short range fighting. It could also be used as a throwing weapon.[1] During the Chinese Han Dynasty (206 B.C.-221 A.D., 漢朝), the dagger was a secondary defensive weapon, and all of the soldiers were required to carry it. Daggers were usually carried in a pair.

Zi Wu Mandarin Duck Axe, Deer Hook Sword or Deer Antler Saber (Yuan-Yang Yue or Lu Jiao Dao, 鴛鴦鉞、鹿角刀**) (Figure 3-13).** There are many names for this weapon. It was also called "Zi-Wu Mandarin Duck" (Zi-Wu Yuan-Yang Yue, 子午鴛鴦鉞) or "Sun-Moon Heaven-Earth Sword" (R Yue Qian-Kun Jian, 日月乾坤劍). "Zi" means "midnight," which implies "Yin," while "Wu" means "noon," and implies "Yang." Sun and Heaven are also classified as "Yang," while the Moon and Earth are classified as "Yin." This is a special weapon, originating from Baguazhang style. It was said that this weapon was specially designed to defeat

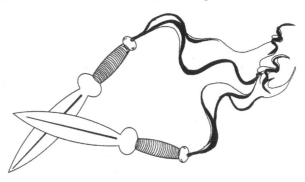

Figure 3-12

the sword. Its shape is like Baguazhang's Yin-Yang fish (Bagua Yin-Yang Yu, 八卦陰陽魚). It was commonly used in a pair, like the male and female mandarin duck which are always together. The weapon is called "Sun-Moon" or "Zi-Wu,"

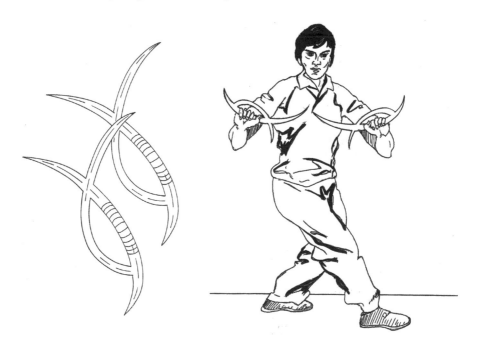

Figure 3-13

55

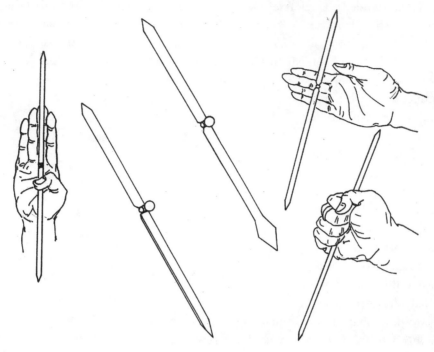

Figure 3-14

because when one manifests its intention (Yang), the other is already prepared for an attack (Yin).

The weapon has been mis-translated in the past as "Deer Hook Sword." However, the correct translation is really "Deer Antler Saber," because of the weapon's resemblance to a stag's antlers. There is a double hook saber and a single hook saber, referring to the number of antler "branches" or blades on the weapon.

Emei Sting (Emei Ci, 峨嵋刺) (Figure 3-14). The Emei Sting was originally called "Emei Needle" (Emei Zhen, 峨嵋針)[2] It consisted of a metal rod, sharp at both ends, with a ring dividing the rod into two sections, one usually slightly longer than the other. There were also some Emei Ci in which the two sides were of equal length. From the name, we can see that this weapon was developed in the Emei mountain area.

The Emei Sting was originally designed as a weapon for underwater fighting, and was usually used in a pair. The Emei Sting was held with the middle finger in the ring for stability. Both stinging and stabbing were possible. It was a rather uncommon weapon, but one that is very easily hidden when strapped to an arm or leg. It was also commonly used as a throwing weapon.

It is said that the Emei Ci was invented during the Song Dynasty (960-1280 A.D., 宋朝) for underwater fighting. In the Qing Dynasty, it was adapted into a throwing weapon, in San Xi Province (山西省).

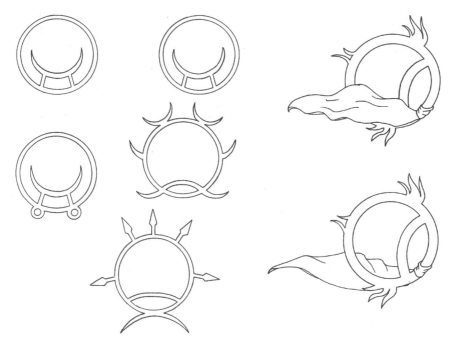

Figure 3-15

Ring or Wheel (Quan or Lun, 圈、輪) (Figure 3-15). Rings or wheels ranged from twelve to eighteen inches in diameter. They were made of metal, and except for the dull grip, the outer edge was sharp. Some rings were unadorned, whereas others had spurs used to block or lock an opponent's weapons and increase the killing potential.

Purely a defensive weapon, the ring served to slide away or block an enemy's weapon. The ring was rarely used, because it could not be easily hidden. If unadorned, the ring slides weapons away. If a ring had spurs, it might be used to lock an adversary's weapon. Rings were commonly used as throwing weapons.

All of these weapons were imported from Mongolia during the Chinese Yuan Dynasty (1206-1368 A.D., 元朝).

Sun-Moon Tooth Saber (R Yue Ya Dao, 日月牙刀) (Figure 3-16). The tooth saber resembles a cymbal that has been cut in half, with a slit in the center for a handle. Both the sun tooth saber and the moon tooth saber are about one and a half Chi across. The two examples shown differ in that the sun tooth saber has sharp teeth along the outer edges whereas the moon tooth saber has only a sharp edge.

Tooth sabers are not easily hidden, and therefore are uncommon weapons. Cutting, sliding or stinging are common techniques, depending on which variety of tooth saber is carried. A martial artist generally carried either two sun tooth sabers or two moon tooth sabers. Rarely would they be mixed.

As with the Ring or Wheel, this kind of saber originated from Mongolia during the Chinese Yuan Dynasty (1206-1368 A.D., 元朝)

Moon Tooth Sting (Yue Ya Ci, 月牙刺) (Figure 3-17). The Moon Tooth Sting is a very short weapon constructed from two spear head-like blades, with a crescent moon saber. This weapon was used in a pair. When this weapon was created is not known. Judging from its shape, it was probably created before the Chinese Song Dynasty (960-1280 A.D. 宋朝).

Palace Heaven Comb (Gong Tian Shu, 宮天梳) (Figure 3-18). This weapon was called a comb simply because it looked like a comb. The four sides are crescent moon-shaped, and the corners are sharp. When and how it was created is unknown. This kind of weapons was popularly used in the Da Yong county of Hunan Province (湖南省，大庸).

Brush (Bi, 筆) (Figure 3-19). The brush or pen was usually made of metal, but could also have been made of bamboo or wood. The metal rod had a sharp metal pen or brush-like head resembling a pen used by judges or scholars. Therefore, it was often called "Judge's Brush" (Pan Guan Bi, 判官筆). More a symbol of justice and scholarship than a martial weapon, the brush was a relatively uncommon weapon. The history of this weapon is unknown. Stabbing is the only effective technique when wielding the brush.

Scissors and Ruler (Jian Dao Chi, 剪刀尺) (Figure 3-20). From the name itself, you can see that scissors and ruler were a tailor's weapon. Both of them were made from metal. How and

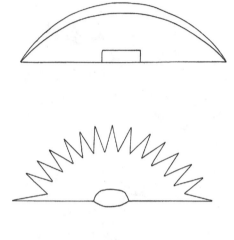

Figure 3-16

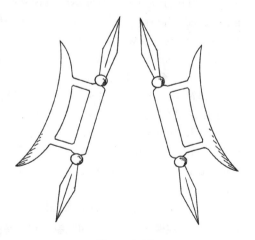

Figure 3-17

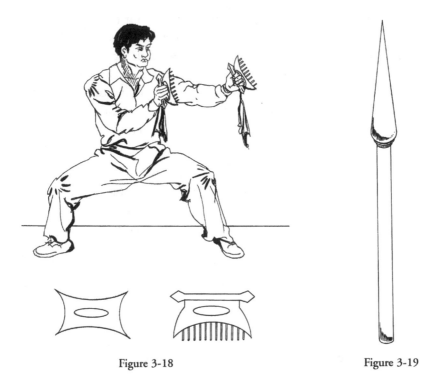

Figure 3-18   Figure 3-19

when they became weapons is unknown. However, these weapons were popularly practiced in Jiangxi Province (江西).[2]

Money Rings and Double Sabers (Qian Ling and Shuang Dao, 錢鈴、雙刀) **(Figure 3-21).** These weapons were also called "Money Thread and Double Saber" (錢串、雙刀). They were popularly used by the Li tribe (黎族) on the Hainan Island of Guangdong Province (廣東省，海南島). Money rings were made from a section of bamboo about two Chi long. The central empty space was filled with coins. When these weapons were used, they made noise. The double sabers are two short sabers, resembling a cow's ears. These weapons are special weapons used by a specific, isolated tribe in China. When and how they were created is unknown.

3-3. Short Weapons

A martial artist carries a short weapon as his primary defensive weapon. It has the advantage of greater killing potential than a very short weapon, and more complex techniques can be applied. Unlike very short weapons, short weapons are rarely thrown, because no smart martial artist would want to lose his or her major defensive weapon.

Martial society today utilizes only a few of the multitude of short weapons. The saber, sword, whip, bar, staff and hook can be found, but techniques used with other short weapons are rarely taught. The techniques for the saber have always been considered to be the foundation of all short weapons. From this foundation, different techniques were developed following the special design or purpose of the individual weapon. Because short weapons were generally lighter than long weapons, they were often used in a pair in order to increase the utility and defensive potential. In this section, we will first introduce common single short weapons, and follow with some examples of double short weapons.

Single Short Weapons 單短兵

Sword (Jian, 劍) (Figure 3-22). The sword is also commonly translated as "narrow blade sword," because it differs from the saber in that the width of the blade is narrower, both edges are sharp, and the handle and sword blade are always straight. Also, the metal protrusion protecting the hand flares out perpendicular to the blade, instead of being circular or semicircular, as with the saber. Normally, the blade itself is less than 1.5 inches wide, and is sharpened so that the first one-third is extremely sharp, the middle one-third is less sharp and the section nearest the handle is dull.

The two basic swords are the scholar sword (Wen Jian, 文劍), and the martial sword (Wu Jian, 武劍). The scholar sword, also known as the female sword (Ci Jian, 雌劍), is lighter and shorter than the martial or male sword (Xiong Jian,

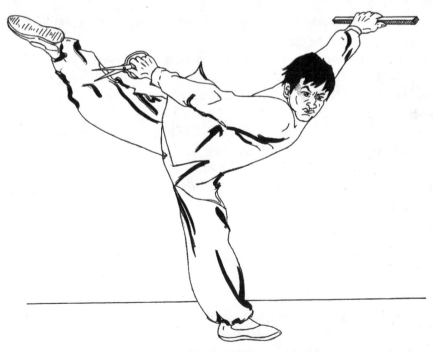

Figure 3-20

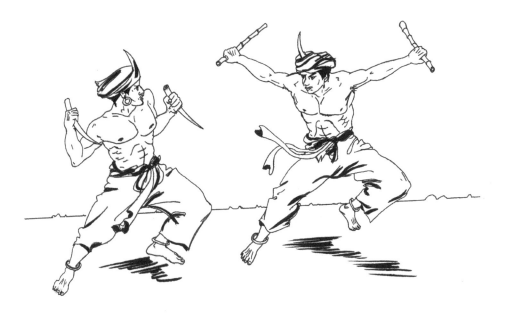

Figure 3-21

雄劍). Another difference lies in the tips of the swords. Whereas the female sword is rounded, the male sword has a sharp tip. In fact, because the martial sword is much heavier than the scholar sword, the martial sword can be used as a battle weapon. However, since the scholar sword is light, and its killing potential relatively weaker than the martial sword, the scholar sword is commonly used as a defensive weapon only.

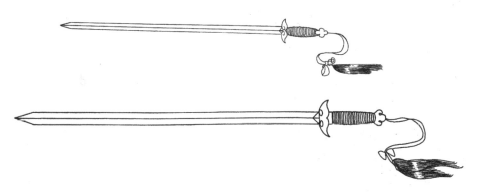

Figure 3-22

During the Chinese Wu Dynasty (222-265 A.D. 吳朝), a hook was added near the tip of the sword to increase the hooking techniques and killing potential (Figure 3-23). Both edges of the hook were sharp. This sword was called "Wu's Hook Sword" (Wu Gou Jian, 吳鉤劍).

There are many other different designs of the sword. Generally speaking, the length of the sword used by the southern martial artists was shorter than that of the northern martial artists. This was because the southern martial artists specialized in short range fighting techniques. Long swords would not be practical for these techniques.

More uncommon swords included the "Snake Head Saw-Tooth Sword" (Ju Chi Jian, 鋸齒劍) (Figure 3-24), the "Snake Tongue Sword" (She She Jian, 蛇舌劍) (Figure 3-25), and the "Wave-Long Sword" (Bo Chang Jian, 波長劍) (Figure 3-26). The serrated edges of the first kind gave it the appearance of a saw blade. Two small holes near the tip resembled the eyes of a snake, and made a whooshing noise when the sword was swung. The second sword had a curved blade, with two sharp prongs instead of a single, pointed tip. The third sword had a wave-like blade to increase its sliding power.

Martial artists considered the sword to be the most versatile of all ancient weapons, and called it the "king of short weapons" (Duan Bing Zhi Wang, 短兵之王). The sharp, upper third of the blade was capable of piercing through an enemy's body. The blade could also be used to cut. The snake head saw-tooth blade had a greatly increased cutting potential.

The lower two-thirds of the sword blade was used to block the opponent's weapon. The flared piece at the top of the handle could lock an opponent's blade as well. This differed from the wide blade sword or saber, which was designed to slide the weapon away rather than lock it. The prongs of the snake tongue sword also served to lock the enemy's weapon.

The hook on the Wu Hook Sword was intended to hook and cut the enemy's arms or legs after blocking his weapon. The hook complicates fighting techniques and increases the weapon's killing potential. However, the disadvantage of the hook sword was that it cannot be put into a sheath.

Techniques for sword fighting are very complicated. Complications arise from the amount of leg and body coordination involved in using the sword as the defensive weapon it was designed to be. Ideally, a martial artist resembles a flying phoenix, flying away to avoid an attack. Only by avoiding and blocking do opportunities arise to stab or cut the enemy.

A martial artist often uses two swords. One sword serves to block, while the other one cuts or stabs. The sword originated from the Huang Di Dynasty (2697-2597 B.C., 黃帝). At first, there was only the short and wide blade sword (or dagger), made from stone or jade. When metallurgical advances continued, the

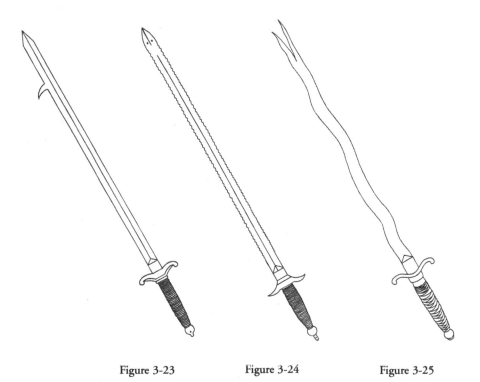

Figure 3-23   Figure 3-24   Figure 3-25

blade was later made from brass, and later with iron. The blade also improved by becoming narrower, longer and sharper.

Saber or Wide Blade Sword (Dao, 刀) (Figure 3-27). The character for saber was also commonly translated as "Wide Blade Sword." The blade was more than 1.5 inches wide, and the handle was often sandwiched between two pieces of wood, and then wrapped with cloth to absorb sweat. A circular or semicircular metal guard protected the hand from an enemy's weapon sliding down the blade. Often, a handkerchief as long as the blade hung from the handle to distract the enemy and to wipe blood off the blade.

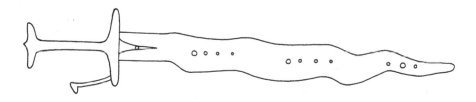

Figure 3-26

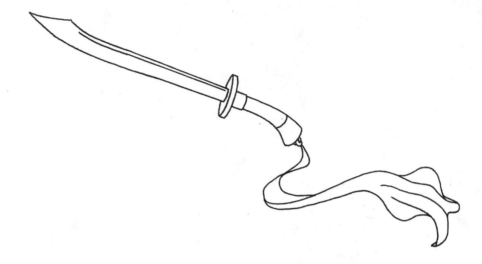

Figure 3-27

Many different types of sabers existed in China. Their structure was dependent on geographic area, martial technique and personal preference. Three structural characteristics were common to almost all sabers. First, the back edge of the blade was dull, except near the tip. Second, the upper one third of the blade was considerably sharper than the lower two-thirds. Finally, each side of the blade had a blood groove.

Sabers favored by Northern Chinese martial artists had curved handles and blades, both to varying extents. These weapons were not very heavy, but they were slightly longer than those used by the Southern Chinese (Figure 3-28). Since the blade of this saber was thin and shaped like a willow leaf, it was called "Willow Leaf Saber" (Liu Ye Dao, 柳葉刀).

The "Goose Feather Saber" (Yan Ling Dao, 雁翎刀) was so named due to its shape, which was like a goose feather (Figure 3-29). This saber was created during the Chinese Song Dynasty (960-1280 A.D., 宋朝).[3] Later, in order to increase the weight to improve killing potential, either the width and the thickness of the blade was increased, rings were installed on the back of the saber, and/or the end of the handle was formed into a ring shape. This design of the saber incorporating all these changes was called "Large Ring Saber" (Da Huan Dao, 大環刀). Different numbers of rings have been used. The most common designs had six rings, called "Six Ring Saber" (Liu Huan Dao, 六環刀) (Figure 3-30) and nine rings, called "Nine Ring Saber" (Jiu Huan Dao, 九環刀).[2] Later, in the Chinese Ming Dynasty

(1368-1644 A.D., 明朝), the design of this saber was again changed into the "Waist Saber" (Yao Dao, 腰刀), in which the blade was thin and long, and the back of the saber was smoothly curved from the handle to the tip (Figure 3-31).[2,5]

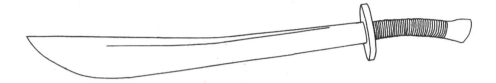

Figure 3-28

Many similar sabers were also created, such as the "Cave Saber" (Wo Dao, 窩刀) which looks like the Japanese Katana used by the Samurai (Figure 3-32). In fact, the precursor to the Katana was imported to Japan from China during the Chinese Song Dynasty (960-1280 A.D., 宋朝). This was called the "Chopping the Horse

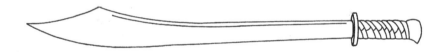

Figure 3-29

Saber" (Zhan Ma Dao, 斬馬刀) (Figure 3-33).[6] It was designed for defense against the cavalry, through chopping the horse's legs. The "Chopping the Horse Saber" is also known in modern times as the "Simple Saber" (Pu Dao, 樸刀). The Cave Saber was an officer's weapon in the Qing Dynasty (1644-1912 A.D., 清朝).[2]

Another kind of saber was called "Miao's Saber" (Miao Dao, 苗刀), which became popular during the Ming Dynasty (1368-1644 A.D., 明朝), when

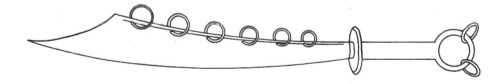

Figure 3-30

Japanese pirates often harassed the Chinese coast (Figure 3-34). The design is very similar to the ones listed in the paragraph above.

Other sabers, such as the "Hand Saber" (Shou Dao, 手刀), were created during the Chinese Song Dynasty (960-1280 A.D., 宋朝) (Figure 3-35). The hand saber was heavier than the other kinds of sabers, and the handle was designed as the handle of a sword.[7] The "Large Chopping Saber" (Da Kan Dao, 大砍刀), was

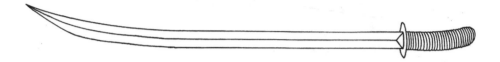

Figure 3-31

heavy and commonly handled with both hands (Figure 3-36). The "Butterfly Saber" (Hu Die Dao, 蝴蝶刀) was short, the blade was wide, and there was an additional hand guard on the handle (Figure 3-37). This was a common southern style weapon, and was commonly used in a pair. When it was used singly, it was usually accompanied by a shield. In fact, most of the lighter sabers were commonly used together with a shield (Figure 3-38).

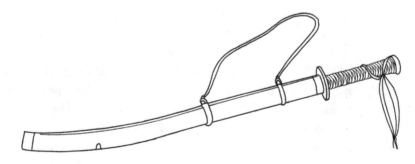

Figure 3-32

The saber is the foundation for all short weapons. The techniques learned for the saber can be applied to all other short arms. As defensive weapons, sabers were most often used for blocking techniques. The dull, back edge of the blade blocks, followed by stabbing or cutting with the sharp edge. The curvature in the blade provides for a violent, powerful repulsion, with less curvature producing less power.

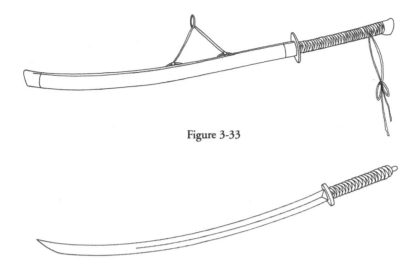

Figure 3-33

Figure 3-34

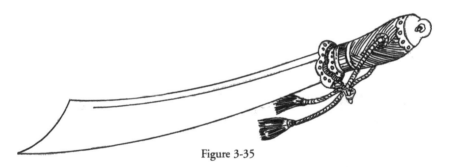

Figure 3-35

Sabers were invented before the Shang Dynasty (1766-1122 B.C., 商朝). During the Chinese Han Dynasty (206 B.C.-221 A.D., 漢朝), sabers were actually straight, and were very different after the Song Dynasty (Figure 3-39).

Whip Rod (Hard Whip) (**Bian Gan,** 鞭桿) **(Figure 3-40).** The whip rod was only a piece of rod as long as a saber or sword. The diameter of one end might be smaller than the other. This was the most ancient weapon, requiring only that a piece of rod be available. Its techniques were a mixture of hard whip and cane. They also included some techniques of the sword and the saber.[8]

Whip (Hard Whip) (Ying Bian, 硬鞭) **(Figure 3-41).** Hard whips are commonly made of hard wood or metal. Sometimes they were made from strong bamboo. The tip of the rod might be either pointed or round, but never sharp. Some whips had hand protectors at the top of the handle. Normally there were joints in the hard whip—the body might be any shape. The joints were shaped to improve killing potential.

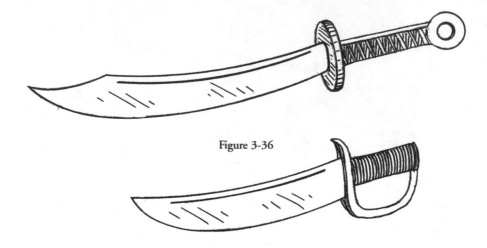

Figure 3-36

Figure 3-37

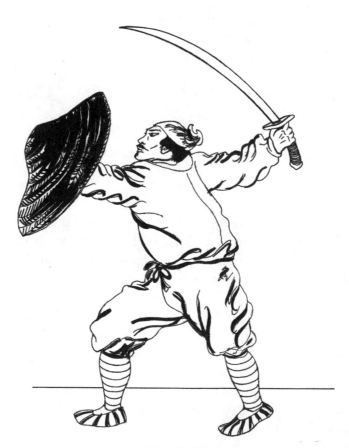

Figure 3-38

The hard whip had little killing potential, and was used by police to subdue offenders. It may have been used to whip a horse. The hard whip could have been used as either a single or double weapon. The single whip was longer and heavier than the double whip.

One of the earliest records of the hard whip comes from the creations of artists of the Song Dynasty (960-1280 A.D., 宋朝).[9, 10] Their renderings of "door gods" show hard whips being carried (Figure 3-42).

Iron Rod (Tie Jian, 鐵鐧、鐵簡) (Figure 3-43). The Iron rod was also called "Iron Slip" (鐵簡), because it was shaped like a "Bamboo Slip," which was used for writing in ancient times. Its shape was like the hard whip, except there were no joints and the tip was not tapered. Moreover the iron rod was shorter and lighter than the hard whip, and therefore was commonly used in a pair, though occasionally it was used singly.

The iron rod was first created during the Chinese Jin Dynasty (265-420 A.D., 晉朝), and it later became more popular in the Tang Dynasty (616-907 A.D., 唐朝). The material used for this weapon during the Jin Dynasty was brass; later it was changed to iron during the Tang Dynasty.[2]

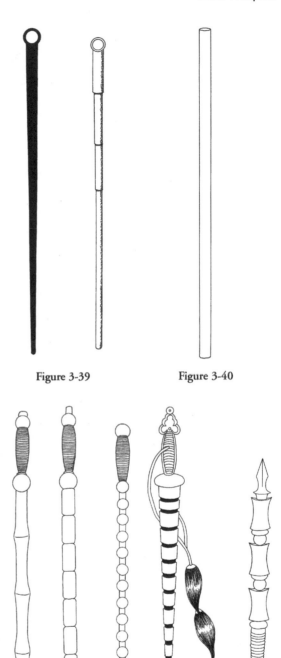

Figure 3-39   Figure 3-40

Figure 3-41

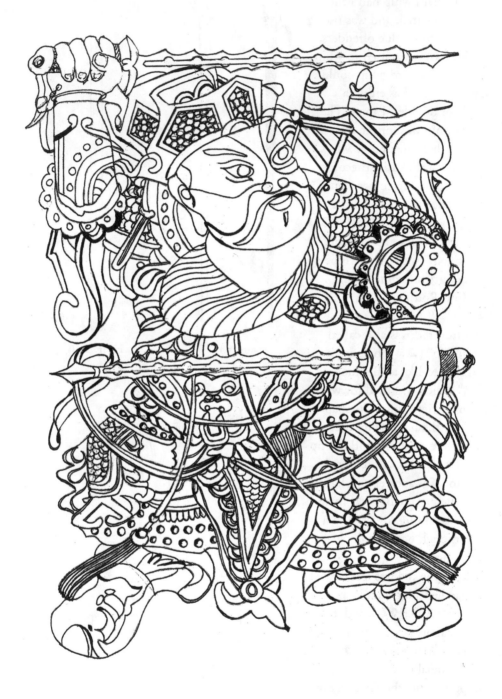

Figure 3-42

Pestle (Chu, 杵) (Figure 3-44). The pestle was made of wood, and was originally used by farmers for cracking rice and other grains. It was also used for striking clothes when cleaning them. Later, the pestle was used to defend against bandits.

Techniques for the pestle resemble those of the short staff, hard whip and iron rod; striking and sweeping are the most common techniques. The pestle dates from Shen Nong (2737 B.C., 神農)

Staff (Bang, 棒) (Figure 3-45). Originally made of wood, and later of metal, the staff was merely a heavy, short rod with a handle. Serrations might cover the rod, as with the wolf's teeth staff, but they are not necessary. Depending on the designs or shape, different names were given.

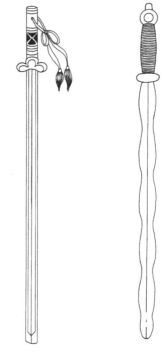

Figure 3-43   Figure 3-44

The staff was originally designed for striking animals. Blocking and then striking are common staff techniques. The heavy staff requires strong arms and wrists. The staff was an ancient weapon with which prehistoric Chinese probably used to hunt.

Short Axe (Fu, 斧) (Figure 3-46). Originally, the axe was comprised of a split stick or club with a piece of stone fixed to it. The axe evolved into a weapon with a sharp, metal head attached to a wooden rod. Different designs or shapes were created and names were also given.

The weight of a short axe made it difficult to block and, therefore, made it an effective weapon for large battles. Chopping, of course, was the main technique of the axe. Occasionally, two axes were carried. Because of the axes' weight, martial artists needed strong arms to wield them. Axes date from before Shen Nong (2737 B.C., 神農).

Crutches (Guai, 拐) (Figure 3-47). The crutch consists of a wooden rod with a peg for a handhold. The crutch originated as an aid for the handicapped. It was easily adapted for martial techniques. The techniques of the crutch resemble those of the long rod except that the handle makes it more effective for sweeping or striking. The crutch probably predates the Spring and Autumn Period and the Warring States Period (722-222 B.C., 春秋戰國).

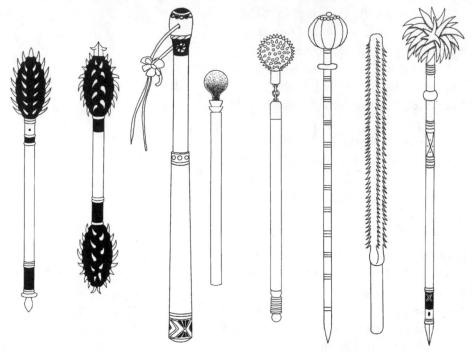

Figure 3-45

Hammer (Chui, 錘、鎚) (Figure 3-48). The hammer resembles the axe except for the head, which was usually rounded, but may be of various shapes. Originally constructed of heavy wood, the later hammers were made of metal. Their original purpose was for construction.

Striking or hitting was the only effective technique for using the hammer. It has little killing potential and remains an impractical weapon. The hammer probably predates Shen Nong (2737 B.C., 神農).

Sword Spear (Jian Qiang, 劍槍) (Figure 3-49). The sharp, double-edged front part of the sword spear was made of metal, whereas the back part was wood. The sword spear was used for short range defense, though it could be thrown. Sliding, cutting and stabbing are all effective techniques. Two sword spears were commonly used at once. The sword spear dates from the Song Dynasty (960-1280 A.D., 宋朝).

Iron Claw (Tie Zhua, 鐵抓) (Figure 3-50). The claw consisted of a wooden handle with a metal head shaped like a hand. The fingers of the hand were very sharp. The iron claw was commonly used in big battles in ancient times. Striking and sweeping were common techniques. Scratching was also effective, because the tips of the fingers were often poisoned. The claw dates from the Han Dynasty (206 B.C.-220 A.D., 漢朝).

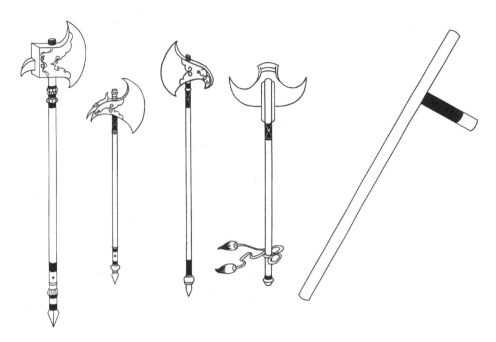

Figure 3-46

Figure 3-47

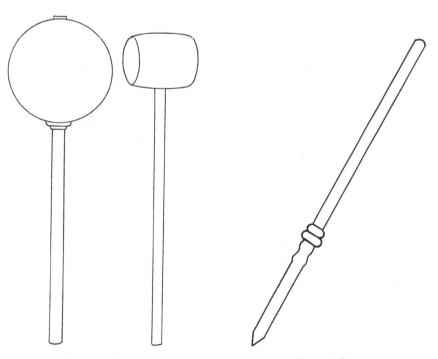

Figure 3-48

Figure 3-49

Blocking Face Pipe (Lan Mian Sou, 攔面叟) (Figure 3-51). This was also called the "Large Smoking Pipe" (Da Yan Dai, 大煙袋) and was made from metal. The length was about 3 feet (110 cm). The blocking face pipe was a special weapon used by the Zhi Zi style (枝子門) of martial arts.[2]

Double Hook Arrow (Shuang Gou Si, 雙鉤矢) (Figure 3-52). The front half of the double hook arrow has a sharp, metal head and two sharp hooks, one on either side of the shaft. The back half of the arrow was made of wood. The hooks of the double hook arrow made it an effective defensive weapon, which could also be thrown. Hooking, stabbing and throwing were all common techniques used with the double hook arrow. The history of this weapon is unknown.

Brass Man (Tong Ren, 銅人) (Figure 3-53). Standing less than three feet tall, the brass man was made entirely of brass and, therefore, was extremely heavy. Priests designed the brass man to strengthen wrists and arms.

When the brass man was used as a weapon, it was grasped around the ankles with one hand and swung. The brass man dates from the Song Dynasty (960-1280 A.D., 宋朝).

Fierce Pincers (Lie Qian, 烈鉆、烈鉗) (Finger 3-54). The history of this weapon can be traced back to the Song Dynasty (960-1280 A.D., 宋朝).[11] One end was fixed with a spear head as long as one and half Chi, and the handle was

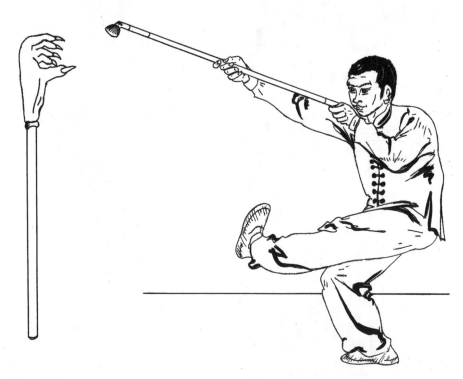

Figure 3-50   Figure 3-51

about three Chi. The bottom had pincers. The details of this weapon are unknown.

Double Short Weapons 雙短兵

As explained in the last section, many of the single short weapons were also commonly used as double weapons, especially those short weapons which were not heavy. The advantage of the double short weapon was the techniques could be more flexible, providing greater killing potential in a fight. The key was using one weapon to block and one weapon to attack. The disadvantage of using double short weapons was that the fighting range was short and ineffective for long range fighting. When double short weapons were used against a long weapon, defense would have precedence over offense. However, if the opportunity arose, one of the double short weapons could become a thrown weapon, reaching to the long range. Yet if the weapon missed the opponent, it was lost, and then the danger was doubled. Next, we will introduce some typical double short weapons.

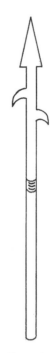

Figure 3-52

Double Sword (Shuang Jian, 雙劍) (Figure 3-55). The double sword was one of the most common double short weapons. The length of the double sword used by northern martial artists was relatively longer than that of the double sword used by southern martial artists. Naturally, the fighting range was also relatively different. The fighting range for northern styles was longer than that of the southern styles. For other details, please refer to the section on the single sword.

Double Saber (Shuang Dao, 雙刀) (Figure 3-56). The double saber was another common double short weapon. The length of the double saber used by northern martial artists was relatively longer than

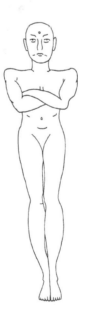

Figure 3-53

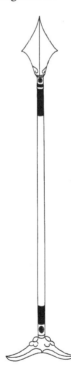

Figure 3-54

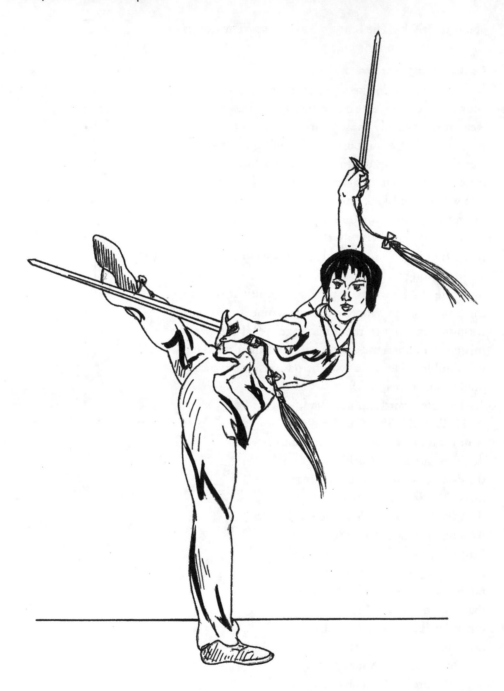

Figure 3-55

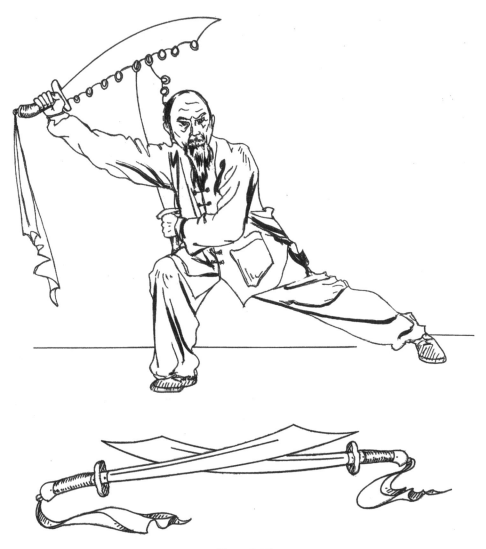

Figure 3-56

that of the double saber used by southern martial artists. Naturally, the fighting range was also relatively different. The fighting range for northern styles was longer than that of the southern styles. For other details, please refer to the section on the single saber.

Butterfly Saber (Hu Die Dao, 蝴蝶刀**) (Figure 3-57).** The butterfly saber was also called "Son-Mother Saber" (Zo-Mu Dao, 子母刀), "Hand Protection Saber" (Hu Shou Dao, 護手刀), or "Wrap Elbow Saber" (Bao Zhou Dao, 包肘刀). The butterfly saber was a common weapon used by many southern martial styles. Its

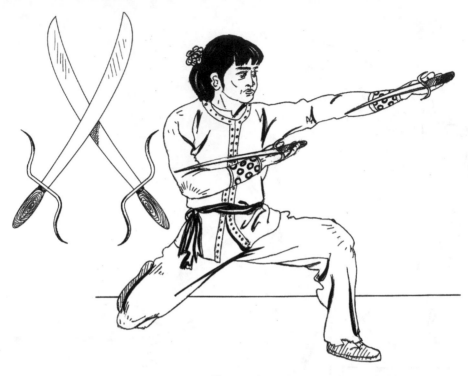

Figure 3-57

range of fighting was short. The saber was able to flip inward and be hidden under the user's elbow and could also be flipped outward and used as a saber. When the butterfly saber was created is unknown, but its design suggests the Ming Dynasty (1368-1644 A.D., 明朝).

Hook (Gou, 鉤) (Figure 3-58). The most common design of the double hook was the "Tiger Head Double Hook" (Hu Tou Shuang Gou, 虎頭雙鉤). The use of the tiger head double hook was similar to that of the hooked sword. It could be used to attack an enemy's or a horse's legs, and it could also be used in personal attacks at very short range. Stabbing, hooking and blocking were all effective, and the crescent over the handle could cut at very close range.

The hook dates from the Spring and Autumn Period and the Warring States Period (722-222 B.C., 春秋戰國).

Double Hard Whip (Shuang Bian, 雙鞭) (Figure 3-59). As explained in the section on single short weapon, the hard whip was commonly used in a pair, and was usually an officer's weapon. Please refer to the section on the hard whip for other details.

Hairpin or Sai (Chai, 釵) (Figure 3-60). The sai was originally a hairpin in ancient times and was later derived into a dagger-like very short weapon, finally

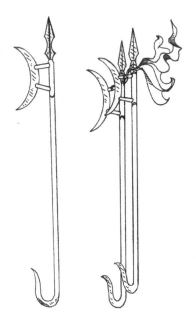
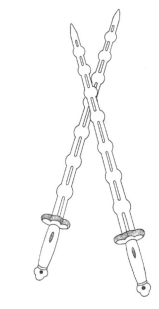

Figure 3-58

Figure 3-59

becoming the sai. The sai consisted of a short, tapered, metal rod, dull at the point, with flared metal prongs guarding the handle. The prongs could be pointed up, or as in the case of the sai used by Southern Chinese, one prong flared upward and the other downward.

The sai was designed for very close fighting, and was predominantly a defensive weapon. It has very little attacking potential. The prongs of the sai, if flared upward, were used to violently block the opponent's weapons. If one prong pointed downward, it was used to parry the enemy's blows. The sai can be used offensively for stabbing, especially the throat, or striking. The shortness of this weapon makes it very easy to rotate it into the arm, and use the metal tip of the handle

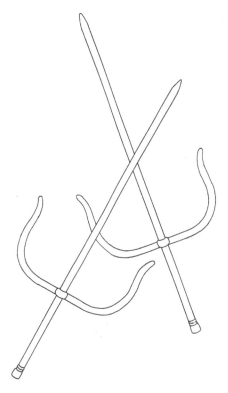

Figure 3-60

for striking at very close range. Often, a martial artist carried two sai. Martial artists in Canton and Fujian Provinces (廣東、福建) favored the sai, as did the Taiwanese (台灣).

The history of the sai's development is unknown. It may date from the Ming Dynasty (1368-1644 A.D., 明朝).

Chicken Claw Yin-Yang Sharp (Ji Zhua Yin Yang Rui, 雞爪陰陽銳 **)** **(Figure 3-61).** This weapon was a special weapon used by Baguazhang style. The structure of the weapon allowed its user to sting, hook, cut and slide. Because one end of this weapon was shaped like a chicken claw, and because it was always used in a pair, it was named "Chicken Claw Yin-Yang Sharp."[8] The techniques for using this

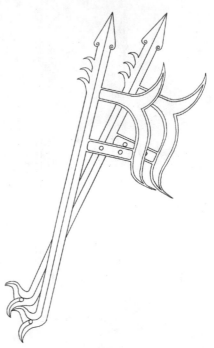

Figure 3-61

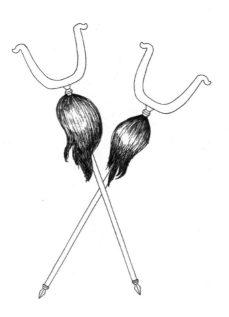

Figure 3-62

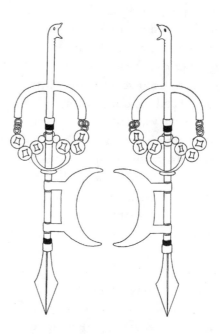

Figure 3-63

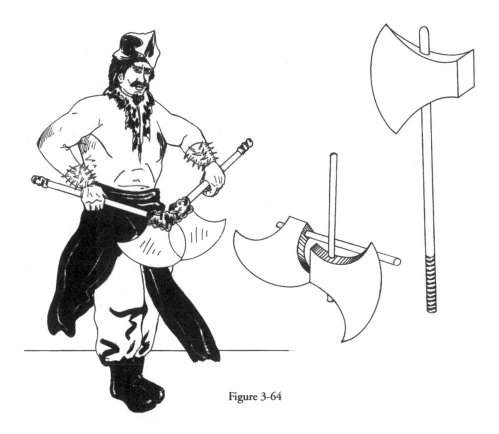

Figure 3-64

weapon were based on the foundation of barehand Baguazhang. The history of using this weapon started in the Qing Dynasty (1644-1912 A.D., 清朝), when Baguazhang was created.

Double Fork Stick (Shuang Cha Gan, 雙叉竿) (Figure 3-62). The double fork stick was derived from the fire fork (火叉). One end of the weapon was a fork, while the other end was fitted with a sharp metal tip. Its major techniques were hooking, poking, twisting, clamping and stinging.[2] The double fork stick may have developed during the Song Dynasty (960-1280 A.D., 宋朝).

Cross Tiger Block (Kua Hu Lan, 跨虎攔) (Figure 3-63). The length of this weapon was about three Chi. It was constructed from a hook, a spear head, and a crescent moon knife. The history of this weapon is unknown.[2]

Double Axes (Shuang Fu, 雙斧) (Figure 3-64). Short axes were commonly used in a pair by those martial artists who had good arm strength. For details on this weapon, please refer to axes in the single short weapon section.

Wolf Tooth Club (Lang Ya Bang, 狼牙棒) (Figure 3-65). The wolf tooth club was usually made from strong wood, and was actually fitted with metal teeth. The

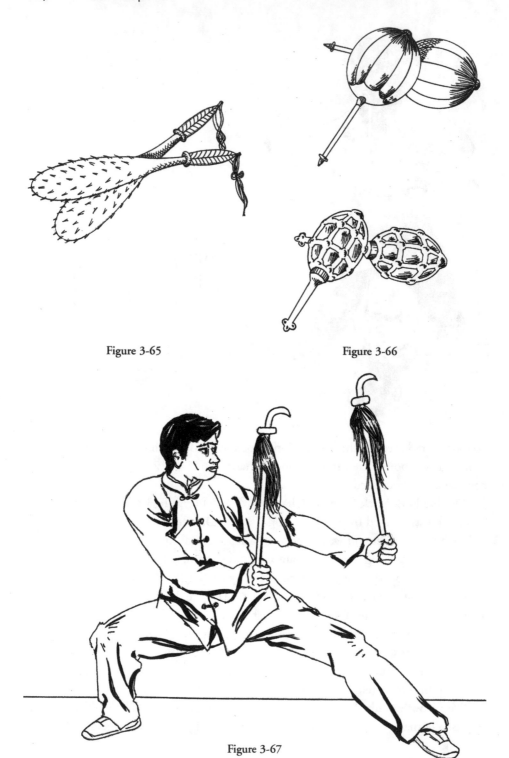

Figure 3-65

Figure 3-66

Figure 3-67

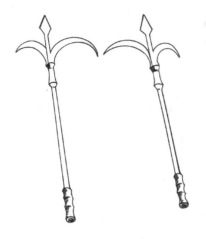

Figure 3-68

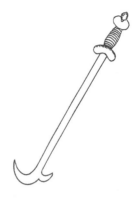

Figure 3-69

weapon was heavy, and therefore, like double axes, needed to be handled by a strong person in battle. Although the killing potential was great, the speed of handling this weapon was too slow for it to become too popular.

Double Hammer (Shuang Chui, 雙錘) (Figure 3-66). The hammer head was normally made from wood or metal, and then fitted with a handle. As with axes and the wolf tooth club, this weapon was heavy and impractical for long battles. Speed was always a problem in handling this weapon.

Blocking Door Pliers (Lan Men Jue, 攔門撅) (Figure 3-67). This kind of weapon was constructed out of a cow horn (or goat horn), or a metal hook which was installed on a length of stick. The length of this weapon was about 3 Chi. Sometimes, it was used as a single short weapon. The details of this weapon are unknown.

Chicken Claw Sickle and Chicken Saber Sickle (Ji Zhua Lian or Ji Dao Lian, 雞爪鐮、雞刀鐮) (Figures 3-68 and 3-69). The chicken claw sickle was constructed from a chicken claw-like piece of metal, along with a spear head, on a length of stick. Its length was about 1.5 feet. The details of this weapon are unknown.

Another similar weapon, the chicken saber sickle, was also called "Binding Flower Waist Carry" (Kun Hua Yao Zi, 捆花腰子). The reason for this optional name is unknown. It is said that this weapon was created by the creator of the "Xin-Yi style" (心意門), Ji, Long-Feng (姬隆丰), and that it became the special weapon of this style. It was made from metal and its length was about 2.5 Chi.[2]

Double Crutches (Shuang Guai, 雙拐) (Figure 3-70). Double crutches are also called "Duckweed Crutches" (Fu Ping Guai, 浮萍拐) or "Sun-Bin Crutches" (孫臏拐). Sun Bin was a well-known martial artist and military strategist during the Spring and Autumn Period and the Warring States Period (722-222 B.C.,

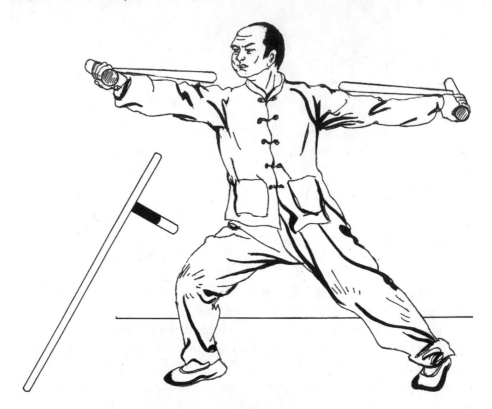

Figure 3-70

春秋戰國). This weapon was popularly
used in the Shanxi Province area
(山西省). Please refer to the section on
crutches for more information.

Horse Halberd (Ma Ji, 馬戟)
(Figure 3-71). The horse halberd was
commonly used in a pair. The length
of this weapon was about 1.5 Chi (40
cm). It was relatively shorter than
other short weapons, and longer than
very short weapons.[2] The details of this
weapon are unknown.

Judge's Brush (Pan Guan Bi,
判官筆) **(Figure 3-72).** The judge's
brush was a special weapon used in
Baguazhang. Occasionally, it was also
used in general martial society.[2] The
history and other details are unknown.

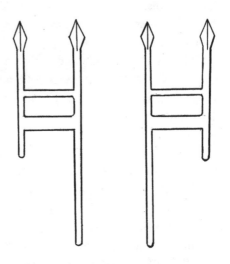

Figure 3-71

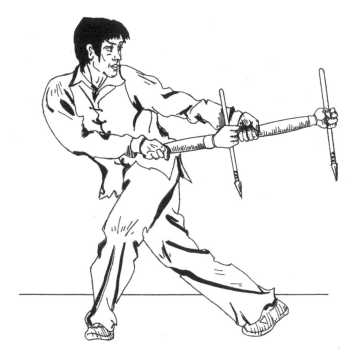

Figure 3-72

Single Dao Crutch (Dan Dao Guai, 單刀拐) (Figure 3-73). Sometimes, two different weapons would be used simultaneously. When this was the case, a martial artist could exploit the advantages of both weapons. For example, when the crutch and the saber were used together, the techniques could be more skillful and more varied. Sometimes, even a soft weapon was used together with a short weapon.

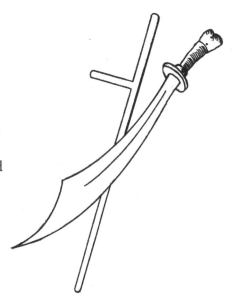

Figure 3-73

References

1. 晉張載《匕首銘》："匕首之設，應速用近，即不忽備，亦無輕念。利以形彰，功以道隱。"

2. *Chinese Wushu Great Dictionary* (〔中國武術大辭典〕，人民體育出版社。1990.

3. 宋王應麟《玉海》卷一五一《兵制》："乾道元年十一月二日，命軍器所造雁翎刀，以三千柄爲一料。"

4. 元張憲《玉笥集》"我有"詩之二："我有雁翎刀，寒光耀冰雪。

5. 明茅元儀《武備志·軍資乘·器械》："腰刀造法，鐵要多煉，用純鋼自背起用平劍平削至刃，刃芒平磨無肩，乃利妙尤在尖。"

6. 《宋史》卷一百九十七《兵制十一》載，斬馬刀"鐔長尺餘，刃三尺餘，首爲大環。"

7. 宋曾公亮《武經總要前集》卷十三《器圖》："手刀一旁刃，柄短如劍。"

8. Zhongguo Wushu,〔中國武術實用大全〕，Kang, Ge-Wu〔康戈武〕，今日中國出版社, 1990.

9. 《宋史·王繼勳傳》："繼勳有武勇，在軍陣，常用鐵鞭，鐵槊，鐵撾，軍中目爲王三鐵。"

10. 明王圻《三才圖繪·器用六卷·兵器類》："鐵鞭鐵簡兩色鞭，其形大小長短隨人力所勝用之。"

11. 宋曾公亮《武經總要》卷十三："烈鑽，刀褥長一尺五寸。上銳，下方闊八寸，柄長三尺，有拐。"

CHAPTER 4

Soft Weapons

軟 兵 器

4-1. INTRODUCTION

Soft weapons include those weapons which were jointed or easily bent. They could be long or short, ranging in length from less than a foot to nearly 30 feet. This chapter will introduce the more common soft weapons. There were also many more individually designed weapons, but it would require too much space to cover all of them.

Soft weapons, with a few exceptions, were primarily secondary weapons, designed for use if the major weapon was lost. They were easily hidden, and because they bend, soft weapons could be stored on the body in such a way as to not interfere with fighting. Usually, the soft weapon was hidden on the waist as a belt (e.g., twelve sectional whip), or strapped to the arm (e.g., chain sword), or on the back (e.g., three sectional whip).

The disadvantages of soft weapons were threefold. First, the techniques involved in their use were difficult to learn. Second, they possessed relatively little killing potential. Finally, soft weapons were easily defended against, especially by an opponent familiar with the weapon. The long rod was most often used in defense, because of its range and ability to wrap around the soft weapon and jerk it from the bearer's grasp.

Many soft weapons can also be classified as thrown weapons. Examples of these weapons, discussed in this chapter include: the comet star hammer (Liu Xing Chui, 流星錘), rope dart (Sheng Biao, 繩鏢) and flying claw (Fei Zhua, 飛爪) etc. They will not be covered again in the chapter concerning thrown weapons.

4-2. SOFT WEAPONS

Sweeper or Broom (Shao Zi, 掃子、梢子) (Figures 4-1 and 4-2). The sweeper can be classified into the large sweeper and the small sweeper. The length of the large sweeper was equal to the martial artist's height. The large sweeper consisted of one long staff connected by chain to a short staff. Each staff was made of hardwood or rattan conditioned with wood-oil.

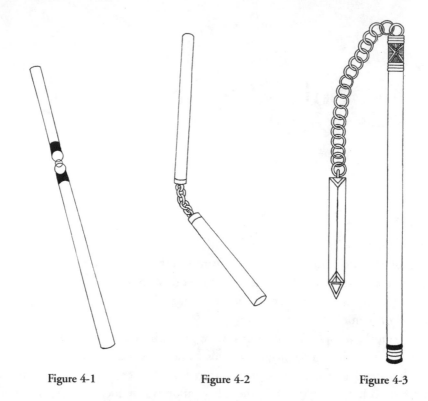

Figure 4-1	Figure 4-2	Figure 4-3

The structure of the small sweeper was the same as the large sweeper, except that each staff was shorter. The small sweeper was more flexible, for shorter striking distances. Small sweepers were commonly used with both hands.

The long, large sweeper was generally used to strike a horse's legs. It could also be effective against a shielded enemy, because the short staff was attached by a chain which bent inward. It was more a disabling than a killing weapon.

By holding the long staff, the martial artist could strike and sweep effectively. The sweeper was difficult to block, because the short staff with its chain was so flexible. It bounced off one block to quickly rebound and strike again.

It is said that the sweeper was invented by the Song emperor Song Taizu (宋太祖), at the beginning of the Song Dynasty (960 A.D.). Song Taizu specialized in the use of the long rod, and one day his favorite rod broke. When he repaired it by chaining the two pieces together, he found it very effective in fighting an enemy bearing a shield, because the short staff could hook over the shield.

Iron Chain Linking Club (Tie Lian Jia Bang, 鐵鏈夾棒) (Figure 4-3). The iron chain linking club was a variation of the sweeper, in which the length of the connecting chain was increased and the short rod was replaced by a sharp, double edged metal head. Sometimes, the metal head would be only a short tapered rod, instead of metal. The increased length of the chain was to increase the sweeping power and therefore, the cutting potential. Moreover, when the metal head was jerked forward, it could act as a speedy projectile spear head. This weapon was probably developed in the same period as the sweeper.

Three Sectional Staff (San Jie Gun, 三節棍) (Figure 4-4). The three sectional staff was constructed from three equal lengths of hardwood or rattan, conditioned with wood-oil and chained together. Its fighting purpose was the same as that of the sweeper, except that the three sectional staff could be used either as a short or a long weapon, depending on which staffs were held.

The techniques for the three sectional staff were more complicated than those of the sweeper. The three sectional staff could be used on either side, and had greater injuring potential. Legend says that Song Taizu later broke his sweeper into three pieces and chained them together.

Soft Hammer (Ruan Chui, 軟錘) (Figure 4-5). The soft hammer was constructed from a comet star maul, to which a short wooden rod was attached by chain. Other than being a battle weapon, the soft hammer was commonly used to build up strength in the arms, shoulders and wrists.

The soft hammer, by virtue of the wooden rod, was not as flexible as other soft weapons. Therefore, the primary techniques used with it were swinging or sweeping. This weapon was developed during the Song Dynasty (960-1280 A.D., 宋朝).

Stick Soft Whip (Gan Zi Bian, 杆子鞭) (Figure 4-6). The stick soft whip was constructed from a piece of stick and a length of rope, to which was attached a metal awl. It is believed that this weapon was derived from the soft whip (西城鞭), popularly used for pasturing sheep in Xiyu (西城). Xiyu is the territory on the western side of China.

From the structure of this weapon, we can see that it could be used as a soft whip, and in addition, when the awl was jerked forward,

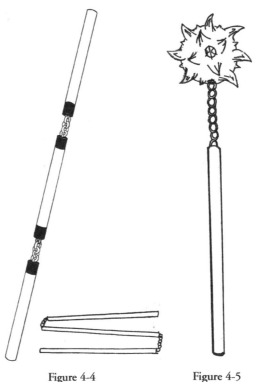

Figure 4-4   Figure 4-5

it could be a powerful projectile weapon. When this weapon was developed is unknown.

Four Sectional Tang (Si Jie Tang, 四節鎲) (Figure 4-7). There is no English translation for the weapon Tang (鎲). It was also called "Tang Lian" (鎲鐮), which means "Tang Sickle." There were four sections. In the first section, there was a snake-shaped blade on both sides, with a sharp tipped, double-edged blade in the front. The other three sections were connected with metal rings. Sometimes, a few hanging, small hammers were connected at the base section. When and how this weapon was created is unknown.

Cangue Staff (Lian Jia Gun, 連枷棍) (Figure 4-8). The cangue staff was originally a farmer's tool which was used for cracking rice and other grains. The cangue

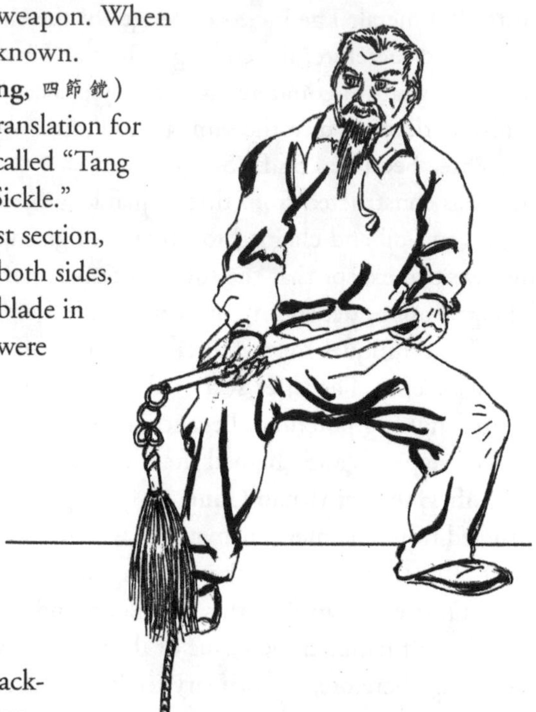

Figure 4-6

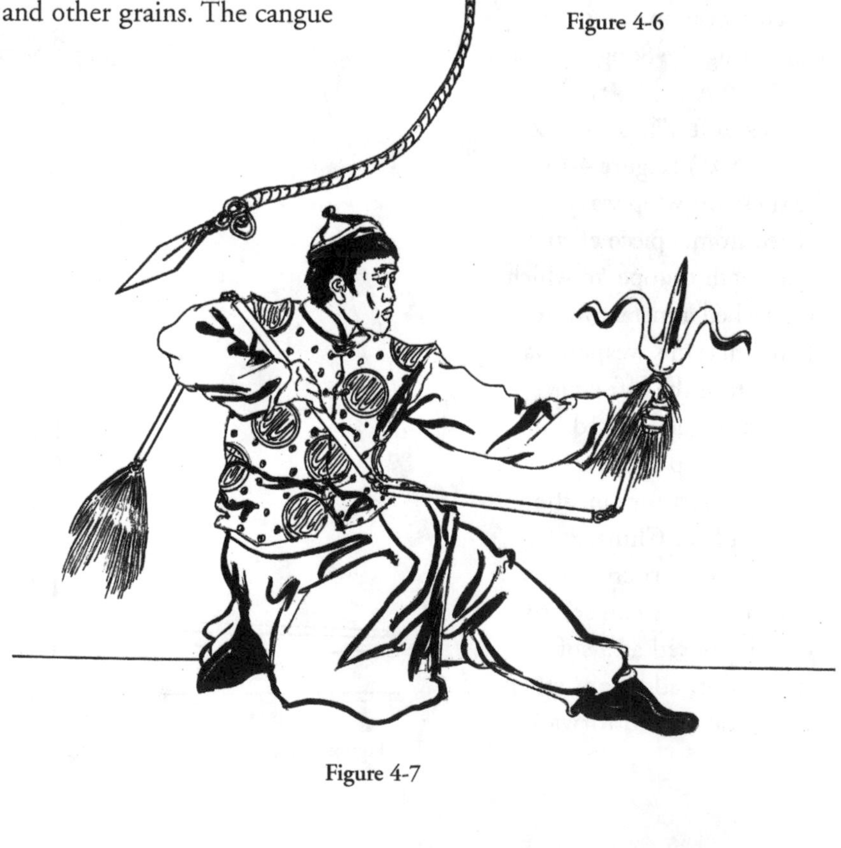

Figure 4-7

staff included a long rod and a short rod, connected with rings or a short chain. When this weapon was imported into Okinawa, the structure varied slightly, and the two connected rods were the same length. This new design was called "Nunchaku," which was translated from the sound of the Chinese word "Lian Jia Gun." As mentioned previously, it was also called "Sweeper" (Shao Zi, 掃子、梢子) in northern China. Therefore, "Lian Jia Gun" was often called "Shao Zi Gun."

This weapon was created during the Chinese Northern Song Dynasty (960-1127 A.D., 北宋). According to available documentation, this weapon was created by Yang Xie (楊偕) during the Song Ren Zong era (1023-1064 A.D., 宋仁宗) and was recommended to the emperor as a military weapon. In its creation, the cangue staff was covered with metal to increase its killing potential, and was called "Fo Lian Jia" (Lian Jia, 鎛連枷).

This weapon was also used in Western China (Xi Xia, 西夏) as a cavalry weapon against foot soldiers. Some ancient documents even claim that the Lian Jia Gun, which was covered with metal, originated from West China. This weapon was used by the Rong tribe (戎人) against Han soldiers during the Chinese Han dynasty (206 B.C.-221 A.D., 漢朝).[1]

Sectional Steel Whip (Jie Bian, 節鞭) **(Figure 4-9).** There were many kinds of sectional steel whips. Common varieties included three, five, seven, nine, ten or twelve steel bars chained together, with a wood or metal handle and a sharp metal head. Usually, the total length of the whip was equal to the user's height. Therefore the length of each steel bar depended on the number of bars; the fewer, the longer.

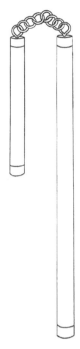

Figure 4-8

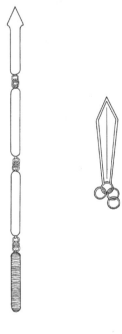
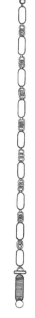

Figure 4-9

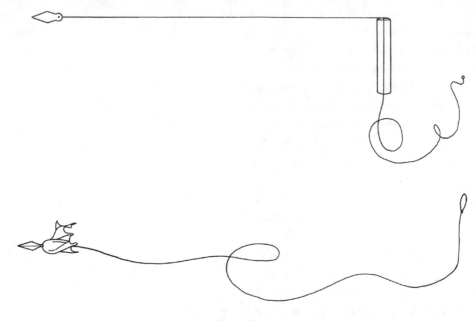

Figure 4-10

Because the sectional steel whip was very flexible, it could be easily hidden. It could be used effectively at long or short ranges, depending on which bar was gripped. It was exceptionally dangerous if the opponent was unfamiliar with it.

The sectional steel whip (except for one with only three sections) could be manipulated with the elbow, knee, foot or neck, and therefore the techniques were innumerable. The whips were best used as stabbing weapons. Sweeping was also a common technique with all whips.

To apply the stab or sweep technique, the steel whip was swung in circles. The direction of the rotation restricted the application of the weapon. For example, if the whip was rotating forward and backward, it was simple to stab (or spear) the enemy, but only if he remained in front. If he shifted to the side, the steel whip needed to be slowed and swung in another direction. Also, once the whip was swinging vertically, it was difficult to use a horizontal sweeping technique.

Use of the sectional steel whip began around the time of the Song Dynasty (960-1280 A.D., 宋朝).

Rope Dart (Sheng Biao or Suo Biao, 繩鏢、索鏢) (Figure 4-10). The rope dart consisted of a heavy, sharp metal head which was slightly smaller than a man's hand and attached to a long (up to 25 feet) rope. Often the rope was made of cow tendons. A small loop at the end of the rope was wrapped around the wrist. Commonly, a bamboo or metal tube about six inches long slid up and down the rope, providing a grip for the other hand.

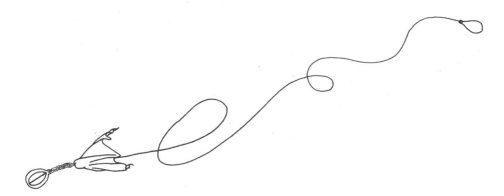

Figure 4-11

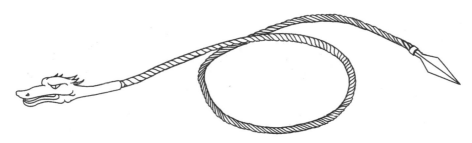

Figure 4-12

The rope dart was almost a throwing weapon, except that it was retrievable. It was easily carried and effective for very long range attacks.

The rope dart, like the steel whip, was rotated around the body to build up speed. It could be directed for stabbing with the elbow, neck, knee or foot. The range of the weapon was controlled by the sliding tube. The rope dart was easily defended against with a long rod or spear. The earliest record of the rope dart is during the Tang Dynasty (618-907 A.D., 唐朝).

Comet Star Hammer (Maul) (Liu Xing Chui, 流星錘) (Figure 4-11). The comet star hammer was also called "Flying Maul" (Fei Chui, 飛錘) or "Long Thread Maul" (Zou Xian Chui, 走線錘). The design of the comet star hammer was very similar to that of the rope dart, except that the sharp, metal head was replaced by a maul. Its application and history are the same as that of the rope dart. Often, mauls were tied up on both ends.

Dragon Head Whip Club (Long Tou Gan Bang, 龍頭杆棒) (Figure 4-12). The dragon head whip club was about six Chi long (nearly six feet). One end had a handle fashioned as a dragon head, and the other end connected to a sharp metal head. Between was a piece of strong, soft rope. Because of its length, it could be used to whip, sweep, wrap, strike, or even sting. Details of the history of this weapon are unknown.

Plum Flower Claw and Dragon Claw (Mei Zha and Long Zha, 梅吒、龍吒) **(Figure 4-13).** The plum flower claw and dragon claw were very similar to the comet star hammer. The difference between these two weapons was that the end of the comet star hammer was a maul, while the plum flower claw and the dragon claw was a claw. Although the look and design of these two claws were slightly different, their application and purpose were the same. They were all used to grab and hook the opponent and pull him down from horse back or higher ground during battle. Often, the claw was poisoned.

Flying Claw or Flying Hook (Fei Zhua and Fei Gou, 飛抓、飛鉤) (Figure 4-14). The flying claw or flying hook resembled the plum flower claw and dragon claw. In the flying claw, the claw was slightly larger than a man's head, and the sharp "fingers" were often poisoned. The fingers were flexible so that once something was hooked it was very difficult to escape the grip.

For the flying hook, the hooks were made from metal, and were hooked inward like a fishing hook. The flying claw or flying hook was an uncommon weapon, but was widely used as a grappling hook to enter buildings, or in a surprise attack against a fleeing enemy. As a weapon, the flying claw was ineffective,

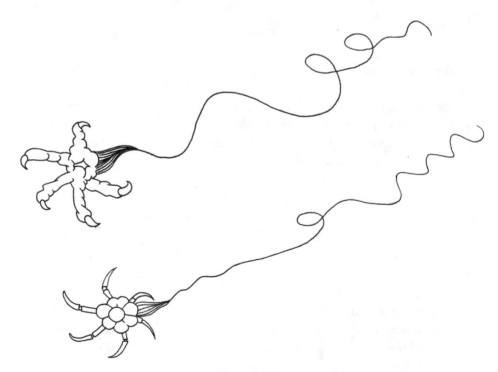

Figure 4-13

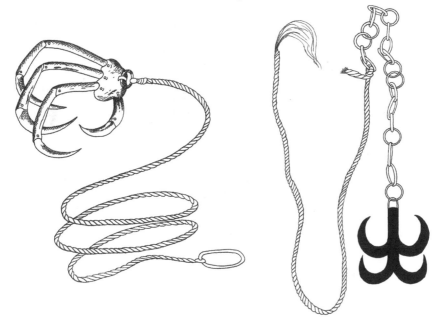

Figure 4-14

except when the points of the fingers were poisoned. There were three other kinds of similar weapons:

1. The Dragon Beard Hook (Long Xu Gou, 龍鬚鉤), which originated in the Song Dynasty (960-1280 A.D., 宋朝).
2. The Rope Hook (Jin Tao Suo, 錦套索), which originated in the Ming Dynasty (1368-1644 A.D., 明朝).
3. The Iron Lotus Flower (Tie Lian Hua, 鐵蓮花), which originated in the Ming Dynasty (1368-1644 A.D., 明朝).

The flying claw and the flying hook originated in the Sui Dynasty (581-618 A.D., 隋朝) and became popular during the Song Dynasty (960-1280 A.D., 宋朝).

Leather Soft Whip (Pi Bian, 皮鞭) (Figure 4-15). The whip was commonly woven from horse or cow leather, which was subsequently immersed in wood oil to increase its endurance and strength. The whip could also be made from the tendons of a cow. Once dried and conditioned, the tendons were much stronger and resistant to cutting than leather. In either case, the whip was attached to a handle of either leather, or wood wrapped with leather. The total length of the whip might reach 12 feet.

The whip was originally designed in Northern China for whipping chariot horses. It was predominantly a defensive weapon. Wrapping and jerking an enemy's weapon away was the most common technique. It might also be used to

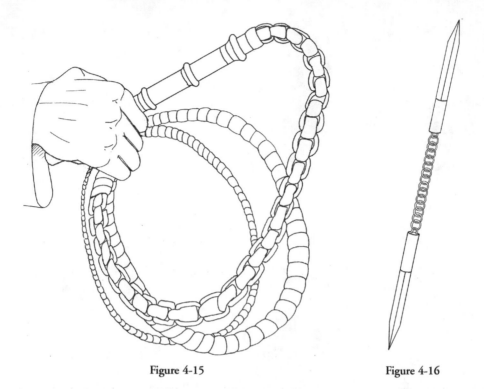

Figure 4-15   Figure 4-16

wrap an opponent's arms or legs to disable him. The whip had almost no killing potential and was ineffective at short range. For these reasons, a dagger was often hidden in the handle.

The whip possibly originated at the time of the Huang Di Dynasty (2697-2597 B.C., 黃帝), contemporaneously to the chariot.

Chain Sword or Chain Brush (Lian Zi Jian or Lian Zi Qiang, 鍊子劍、鍊子筆) (Figure 4-16). The chain sword or brush was constructed from two short daggers or metal brushes, each the length of the user's arm, which were chained together. This was an easily hidden weapon. The chain sword or brush was used as a short-range weapon. The dagger or brush on either side could be easily detached for throwing.

The chain sword or brush could cut, stab or slide. In addition, the base of each dagger or brush could be held so that the chain could be used to block an opponent's weapon. The techniques were difficult to learn, and the chain sword was overall an ineffective weapon. The chain sword originated in the Song Dynasty (960-1280 A.D., 宋朝).

Whip Spear or Chain Spear (Bian Zi Qiang or Lian Zi Qiang, 鞭子槍、鍊子槍) (Figure 4-17). The whip spear was constructed from twelve or more steel rods which were chained together with metal spear heads at each end.

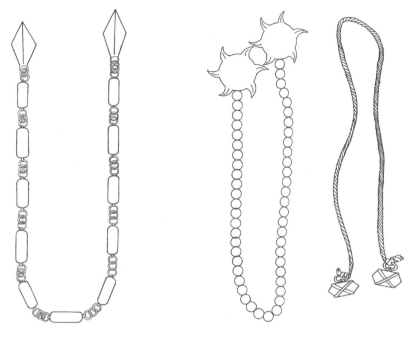

Figure 4-17   Figure 4-18

The length of the whip spear was usually much greater than the user's body. The length of the whip spear and its construction improved both its long and short range fighting potential, compared to the sectional steel whip introduced earlier.

The techniques were more difficult than those for the sectional steel whip, but the whip spear had greater killing potential because of its range and the two spear heads. It was a better weapon than the steel whip at short range, but had the same inherent problem of requiring rotation about the body for longer range attacks. This weapon might have been created during the Song Dynasty (960-1280 A.D., 宋朝).

Double Head Comet Star Hammer or Double Head Flying Maul (Shuang Tou Liu Xing Chui or Shuang Tou Fei Chui) (雙頭流星錘、雙頭飛錘) (**Figure 4-18**). The double head comet star hammer or flying maul was very similar to the single head comet star hammer or maul introduced earlier, except that there were two metal heads or mauls connected by a long chain or rope. Normally, one hammer was thrown at the opponent, and the other was held to prepare for the second attack.[2]

Often, a small ball hammer was swung and thrown toward a horse's legs to tumble its rider to the ground. This weapon probably originated in Tibet during the Tang Dynasty (618-907 A.D., 唐朝).

Double Flying Claw (Shuang Fei Zhua, 雙飛撾) (Figure 4-19). The double flying claw was very similar to the single flying claw, except that there was one claw attached at each end of the rope. The fingers were flexible so that once something was hooked it was very difficult to escape the grip. Normally, one end was thrown toward the enemy, while the other end was held ready for a second attack if the first attack missed. This weapon was commonly used against cavalry.

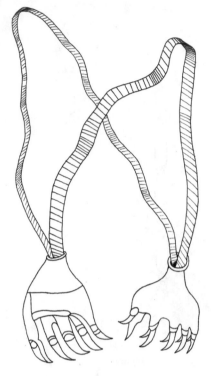

Figure 4-19

References

1. 《武經總要前集》卷十三《器圖》：〝鐵連枷棒本出西戎，馬上用之，以敵漢之步兵，其狀如農家打夗之枷，以鐵飾之，利于自上擊下，故漢兵善用者巧于戎人。〞

2. 《武備志‧器械》載：〝飛錘即流星錘也。錘有二，前者爲正錘，后面手中握者爲之救命錘。〞

3. 明茅元儀《武備志》卷一百零四《軍資乘‧器械》雙飛撾：〝用淨鐵照樣式打造鷹爪樣，五指攢中，釘活，穿長繩系之，始擊人馬，用大力人丟去，著身收合，回頭不能脫走。〞

CHAPTER 5

Projectile and Throwing Weapons

投射兵器

5-1. INTRODUCTION

Projectile and throwing weapons differ from most other Chinese weapons because they have no defensive capabilities: they were designed solely for attack at long or short ranges. These weapons could be projected by throwing, spitting, or firing from a string or a spring. In each case, the weapon, once used, was not recoverable. If it missed its mark, the weapon could then be utilized by the enemy.

This trait of non-retrievability differentiates throwing weapons from various soft weapons that could also be thrown. The rope dart (Suo Biao or Sheng Biao, 索鏢、繩鏢), comet star hammer (Liu Xing Chui, 流星錘), and flying claw (Fei Zhua, 飛爪) could all be thrown but remained attached to the arm by a rope.

Other weapons could be classified as throwing weapons but seem better suited to being categorized with previously discussed groups of weapons. The daggers (Bi Shou, 匕首), Emei Sting (Emei Ci, 峨嵋刺), cymbals (Ba or Nao, 鈸、鐃), scrape saber (Xiou Dao, 削刀), short sword (Duan Jian, 短劍), short saber (Duan Dao, 短刀), short trident (Duan Cha, 短叉), and ring (Lun or Quan, 輪、圈) could be thrown but were better classified as short or very short weapons. The long weapons spear (Qiang, 槍) and trident (Cha, 叉) might also be classified as throwing weapons, but have been discussed previously.

The only throwing weapons covered in this chapter are those designed for personal use. Devices that require gun powder or other non-human means for projection, such as rocket arrows, are excluded.

5-2. PROJECTILE AND THROWN WEAPONS

Bow and Arrow (Gong Jian, 弓箭) (Figure 5-1). The ancient Chinese bow and arrows resemble those of Western cultures. The bow was originally made of bamboo, then of stronger and more flexible wood, and finally of metal. Arrows were constructed from the same materials. Cow tendons, deer skin, silk, or cotton thread served as strings.

Bows and arrows were most often used as an initial attacking weapon in large battles. Only rarely did one utilize a bow and arrow in personal fighting. In fact, the original purpose of the bow and arrow was to hunt animals for food. Therefore, the use of the bow and arrow might have originated even before the Huang Di Dynasty (2697-2597 B.C., 黄帝).

Sling Bow or Sling Shot (Dan Gong, 彈弓) (Figure 5-2) There were three kinds of sling shots or sling bows in ancient times. The first kind was constructed from a "Y" shaped branch, which was very similar to today's sling shot. The only difference was that, because in ancient times there was no rubber to make a string that was as elastic as today the string was made from tendons and an elastic wood was chosen.

The second kind was the sling bow, which resembled a bow and arrow, except that an iron ball replaced the arrow, and a leather pouch was installed on the string for firing. The third kind was the sling shot, which somewhat resembled a crossbow in which the metal ball was placed on the chute and then fired.

The sling bow and sling shot were commonly used as individual weapons for surprise attacks. They

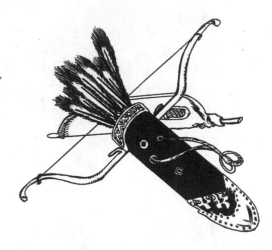

Figure 5-1

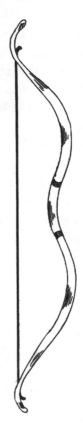

Figure 5-2

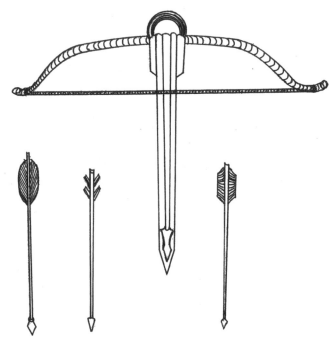

Figure 5-3

were seldom used for big battles. The reason for this was because they did not have as great a killing potential as the bow and arrow.

The balls for the sling bow and sling shot were commonly made from dirt which had been dried or baked. The dirt was later mixed with metal powder, in order to increase its weight. Finally, brass or iron balls were used to increase the injury potential.

Crossbow (Nu, 弩) (Figure 5-3). The crossbow was made from the same materials, and resembled the Western crossbow. The Chinese crossbow, however, was capable of firing three, four or five arrows simultaneously. On the bow, there was a special design which included the hook (Gou, 鉤; ancient name: Ya, 牙), scope (Zhao Men, 照門; ancient name: Gui, 規), and trigger (Ban Ji, 扳機; ancient name: Xuan Dao, 懸刀).

There were many kinds of crossbows. The kind that could be opened with the arms was called "Arm Open Crossbow" (Bi Zhang Nu, 臂張弩). Those that needed a foot in order to be opened were called "Foot Open Crossbow" (Jue Zhang Nu or Ta Zhang Nu, 蹶張弩·踏張弩). If they required waist power to open, they were called "Waist Open Crossbow" (Yao Zhang Nu, 腰張弩). Those large and long distance ones that needed many people to open them by using a gear or capstan were called "Bed Crossbow" (Chuang Nu, 床弩), since the crossbow was

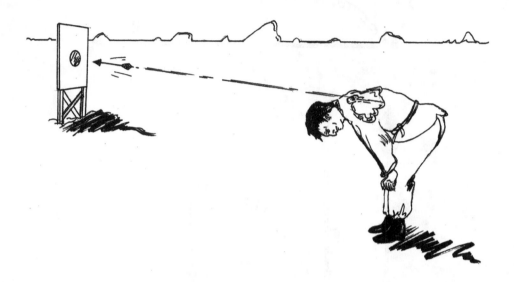

Figure 5-4

installed on a specially designed, movable bed. Finally, those that needed a specially designed capstan were called "Car Crossbow" (Che Nu, 車弩).

The advantage of the crossbow was that it was more powerful, so that it could reach longer distances. It could also be aimed more accurately than the bow and arrow. However, its operating speed was slower than the bow and arrow. Because of this, the crossbow was rarely used in personal fighting, but only for big army battles in ancient times.

Back Crossbow (Bei Nu or Hua Zhuang Gong, 背弩、花裝弓) (Figure 5-4). The back crossbow was spring-loaded, in a tube, and strapped to the back. Triggering occurred upon bowing. The length of the arrow was about 1.5 to 2 Chi. The design of the back crossbow was very similar to the sleeve arrow, which will be discussed later. Back crossbows were effective in surprise attacks at distances of up to 30 steps. The power and killing potential of a back arrow was much stronger than that of the sleeve arrow. It is said that the back crossbow was invented by Xu, Liang-Chen (徐亮臣) in the Northern Song Dynasty (960-1127 A.D., 北宋).

Step Crossbow (Ta Nu, 踏弩) (Figure 5-5). The step crossbow was identical to the back crossbow, except for being slightly shorter (2/3 to 1 Chi). It was hidden in the sole of the shoe or in the stirrup of a saddle. The arrow was shot

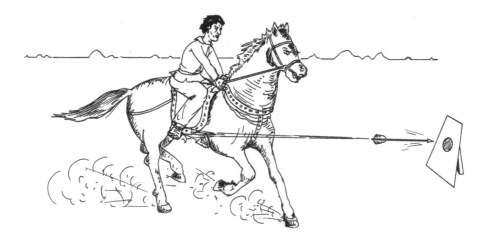

Figure 5-5

from a tube by stepping on a release
button. The step crossbow was used in
surprise attacks against both humans and
their horses. It is believed that Xu,
Liang-Chen (徐亮臣) invented this
weapon during the Northern Song
Dynasty (960-1127 A.D. 北宋).

**Flying Darts (Fei Biao, 飛鏢) (Figure
5-6).** Hundreds of individually designed
darts exist: only one example is provided
for purposes of brevity. The forward part
of the dart had two sharp edges and a
very sharp point, whereas the rear por-
tion was dull. Often, a cloth was
attached to the small ring on the back
for stabilization. Sharp stones originally
served as darts.

Darts were effective up to about 10
to 20 steps. They had no defensive purposes whatsoever. Good martial artists
were able to throw up to five darts at one
time accurately.

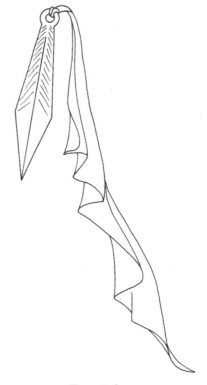

Figure 5-6

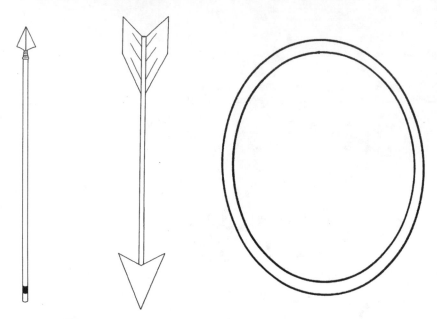

Figure 5-7

Figure 5-8

According to legend, during the Northern Song Dynasty (960-1127 A.D., 北宋), the priest Xing Yuan (性圓) traveled to Tibet and learned the techniques of the dart, then bringing the weapon back to China.

Throwing Arrows (Shuai Shou Jian, 摔手箭) (Figure 5-7). Throwing arrows were slightly larger than, but otherwise identical to, sleeve arrows which will be discussed later. As the name implies, throwing arrows were thrown, not spring-activated like sleeve arrows. Throwing arrows were easily hidden and were useful in surprise attacks at slightly greater range than sleeve arrows.

Throwing arrows were thrown like spears or swung from the side of the body. Throwing arrows developed with the bow and arrow in the Huang Di Dynasty (2697-2597 B.C., 黃帝).

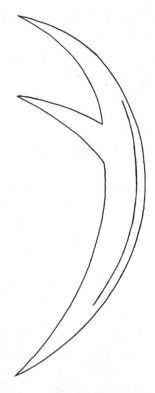

Figure 5-9

Sleeve Ring (Xiu Quan, 袖圈) (Figure 5-8). Any metal bracelet with dull edges could serve as a sleeve ring. Sleeve rings were effective for distracting an enemy at very short range. They were commonly used to throw in an enemy's face for minor injury.

Sleeve rings could be tossed in a disc-like manner or thrown. Sleeve rings were popular ornaments and date from at least Yuan Dynasty (1206-1368 A.D., 元朝).

Dart Knife (Biao Dao, 镖刀) (Figure 5-9). The dart knife consisted of a curved metal blade with a bifurcated end. All edges and points were sharp, but the longer part of the blade, which was used for throwing, was less sharp. Dart knives might have originally been carved from wood.

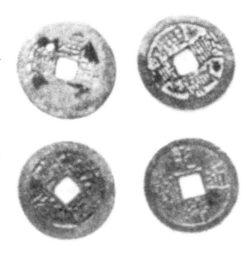

Figure 5-10

The dart knife, because of its sharp edges, had good killing potential, and could be thrown in attack to lengths of up to 30 steps. The dart knife was most often thrown at the enemy's throat. Because of the curved blade, the dart knife could be thrown in a curve, and so was not restricted to direct frontal attack.

The dart knife did not originate in China. It was probably imported from Tibet.

Lo Han Coins or Throwing Coins (Luo Han Qian or Zhi Qian, 羅漢錢、擲錢) (Figure 5-10). Any ancient or modern coins could serve as a Lo Han coin. The examples given have center holes, but they were not necessary. Coins were often carried in an easily reachable pocket, providing a simple, surprise weapon.

When coins were used for attack, they were tossed or flipped, held either with the thumb and first finger or with two fingers. Often, many coins were thrown at the enemy's face. The edges were sharpened but never poisoned, because of the danger of self-inflicted wounds. Usually, it took three years of practice to master the techniques of Lo Han coins. The final test of ability was to be able to penetrate a watermelon with one coin.

Martial artists probably utilized coins in self-defense since their invention.

Mother-Son Cross Dart (Mu-Zi Shi Zi Biao, 母子十字鏢) (Figure 5-11). The star-like cross dart was made entirely of metal and was the size of the palm or slightly smaller. Only one edge of each of the four points was sharp. Cross darts were effective at medium range (10 to 20 steps). They could be tossed like a disc or thrown from the side of the ears. Cross darts date from the Northern Song Dynasty (960-1127 A.D., 北宋). It is possible that when Chinese culture was imported into Japan, the cross dart also became a Japanese martial weapon. The Tang and Song Dynasties were the two dynasties which greatly influenced Japanese culture.

Sleeve Arrow (Xiu Jian, 袖箭) (Figure 5-12). The sleeve arrow resembles an arrow used with a bow. It had a bamboo shaft with or without tail feathers, and a pointed metal head. The sleeve arrow was spring-loaded in a tube, strapped to the arm and released by a string attached to the fingers. Occasionally, five arrows might be fired from a single tube. Such a weapon was called "Plum Flower Sleeve Arrow" (Mei Hua Xiu Jian, 梅花袖箭), because it resembled the five petals of a plum flower.

Surprise attack at close range (five to ten steps) was the primary use of the sleeve arrow. Because the sleeve arrow had little power, it could not penetrate thick clothing. Therefore, the tip was often poisoned and aimed at the face of an adversary. Sleeve arrows were invented during the Northern Song Dynasty (960-1127 A.D., 北宋).

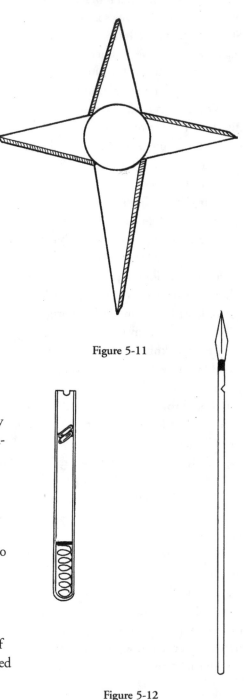

Figure 5-11

Figure 5-12

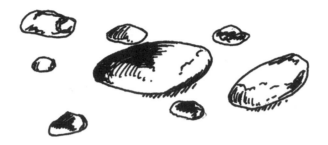

Figure 5-13

Flying Locust Stones (Fei Huang Shi, 飛蝗石) (Figure 5-13). Any small stones served as flying locust stones. Iron balls (Tie Dan Zi, 鐵彈子) were also considered flying locust stones. Moreover, often a single large stone was also classified as a flying locust stone.

Throwing was the only technique, and its effective distance was very short. The flying locust stone originated when prehistoric man first threw loose stones.

Sleeve Egg (Xiu Dan, 袖蛋) (Figure 5-14). The sleeve egg was very similar to the flying locust stone. The sleeve egg could be stone or metal, and was the size of a bird's egg which could be hidden in the sleeve in ancient Chinese clothing. As with flying locust stones, the sleeve egg was used for short range sudden attacks during a fight.

Flying Sting (Fei Ci, 飛刺) (Figure 5-15). The flying sting was very similar to the sleeve egg. The difference was that both ends of the flying sting were tapered and sharp to increase their injuring potential. Since throwing was the only technique, they could be used only in short range fighting.

Brass Chopsticks (Tong Zhu, 銅箸) (Figure 5-16). Chopsticks have been a daily utensil for eating in China. Although most chopsticks were made from bamboo, chopsticks made from other materials such as brass, silver, gold, and iron were not uncommon in ancient times. When thrown with correct technique and power, it could become a weapon, especially when it was thrown toward the face, since one end of the chopsticks was tapered.

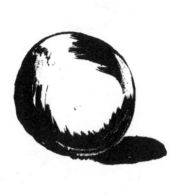

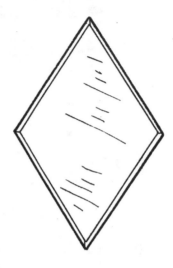

Figure 5-14

Figure 5-15

Iron Mandarin Duck (Tie Yuan Yang, 鐵鴛鴦). The iron mandarin duck was a throwing weapon in which the mandarin shape was made from either brass or iron. It was about the same size as a fist. Compared with other throwing weapons, the iron mandarin duck was heavier and harder to carry.

Plum Flower Needles (Mei Hua Zhen, 梅花針). Plum flower needles resemble the poison darts of certain African tribes. The tail end of a simple sewing needle was wrapped with thread, so that it fit tightly in a small tube made from a feather. Plum flower needles were always poisoned. Often, five needles, resembling the petals of the plum flower, were loaded into a single tube.

The poisoned needle emerging from a tube in the mouth works very well in short-range fighting. The history of this weapon is unknown. It was probably created once metal was available for needle making.

Poison Sand or Red Sand Hand (Du Sha or Hong Sha Shou, 毒砂、紅砂手). Any sand that had been treated with poison could be called poison sand. It was called red sand hand simply because the sand became red colored after the poison treatment. The poison sand was used to attack the enemy's eyes by surprise at

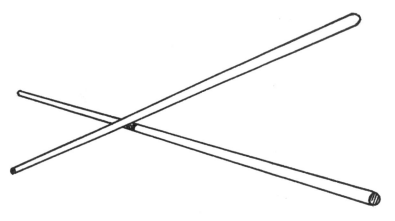

Figure 5-16

short range. The disadvantage of poison sand was that the poison could also affect your own hand.

When poison sand was used in a battle, the thrower needed to keep his back to the wind. If not, the wind might blow the sand into his own eyes. It is believed that poison sand was developed very early in Chinese history. When exactly this was is unknown.

In this chapter, I can only offer the information that I am able to find in existing documents. There were many other aerial weapons. Although the names are recorded, such as "Blood Drop Thrower" (Xue Di Zi, 血滴子), "Iron Lotus Flower" (Tie Lian Hua, 鐵蓮花), etc., exactly how and when they started is unknown. Moreover, the shape, the size, the structure, or the techniques cannot be found.

CHAPTER 6

Shields and Armor

盾牌與鎧甲

6-1. INTRODUCTION

Shields and armor were always considered one of the most important armory designs in ancient military defense. The strength, size, weight and effectiveness of shields and armor were critical factors for securing victory. For example, if a shield or armor was too heavy to carry and to wear, it would not be easy for its user to move quickly and smoothly in battle. This was especially true if the shield and armor were used for cavalry. After many thousands of years of development in ancient times, the common materials used for Chinese armor were rattan or strong wood covered with leather. Metal shields and armor were also used for a period of time in Chinese history. However, due to their weight and the inconvenience of carrying and handling them, their use was abandoned in a short time. It was not until later, when iron was popularly used and metallurgical technology was advanced to a higher level, that metal shields which were thin and strong were developed.

In this chapter, we will review some of the most common designs for the shields and armor used in ancient times. Due to the scarcity of ancient documents, there is only a limited amount of information which can be offered in this chapter.

6-2. SHIELDS

Shields were commonly called "Gan" (block or shield, 干)[1], "Dun Pai" (shield board, 盾牌), "Peng Pai" (big board, 彭牌), or "Pang Pai" (side board, 旁牌)[2] in ancient times (Figure 6-1). They were also customarily called "Dang Jian Pai" (擋箭牌) which means "the blocking arrow shield." This implies that the main purpose of the shield was to block either hand weapons or projectile weapons.

The common shapes of the shield were rectangular or round. Normally, the rectangular shields, which were larger and heavier, were used by foot soldiers, and were called "Bu Dun" (stepping shield or foot soldier's shield, 步盾), while those shields which were lighter and smaller were used by charioteers, and were called "Zi

Dun" (son shield, 子盾). Traditionally, these shields were made from strong wood, and were covered in leather. Later, when cavalry was becoming popular in battle, a specially designed shield for the cavalry was invented. These shields were round, smaller and lighter; they were called "Ji Bing Pang Pai" (cavalry's side shield, 騎兵旁牌).

The rectangular, heavy shield was often held steady on the ground, and the soldiers would duck behind the shield to hide from incoming projectile objects. However, the round and light shields were also commonly used by foot soldiers for face-to-face ground fighting against the enemy. Moreover, the round shields made from rattan, called "Teng Pai" (rattan shield, 藤牌)[3], were used by foot soldiers to chop at enemy cavalry horses' legs.

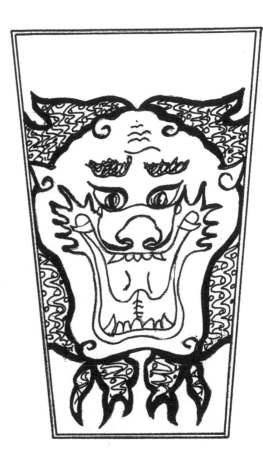

Figure 6-1

It is said that the strategy of using the shield and a hooked sword against cavalry and chariot was created by Marshal Yue Fei (岳飛), during the Chinese Southern Song Dynasty (1127-1280 A.D., 南宋) (Figure 6-2). At this time, the Southern Song were resisting the invasion of the Northern barbarians called "Jin" (金). The most powerful Jin commander, Wu Zhu (兀朮), had never lost a battle. Wu Zhu's terrifying success was largely due to his main weapon — the feared "Guai Zi Ma" (拐子馬). The Guai Zi Ma was an ancient version of the tank. It was a chariot carrying armored men, drawn by three fully armored horses which were connected by a chain. It was extremely difficult to disable either the horses or the riders, and so they completely dominated the battlefield.

Yue Fei had given much thought to defending against the awful Guai Zi Ma. As in other cases, Yue's brilliant military mind came up with a solution. He found that the horses were not protected in one place—their legs. Putting armor on the

horses' legs would have made them
immobile. It was too difficult to attack
the horses' legs with conventional arrows
and spears, so Yue Fei devised two simple
but effective weapons: a sword with a
hooked end, which was extremely sharp
on the inside edge of the hook, and a
shield made out of a vine called "rattan"
(Teng, 藤). Yue Fei's army was called
"Teng Pai Jun" (藤牌軍), or "the rattan
shield army."

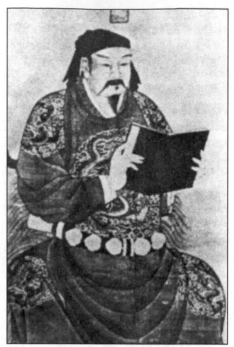

Figure 6-2

At last, both generals met on a fateful
day. When the battle started, Yue Fei had
the Rattan Shield Army crouch very low
in the path of the Guai Zi Ma. Before
the chariots could reach the soldiers, they
ran into obstacles, such as ditches and
upright spears which Yue Fei had set up.
Once these slowed down the chariots,
Yue Fei's soldiers, who were mainly on
foot, could move against the enemy with
more ease. As the chariots advanced, the crouching men hooked and cut the legs
of the horses, making them fall. It was impossible for the horses to trample the
crouching men because the shields were greased, and the horses slipped every
time they put their feet on them. When the crouching soldiers attacked the horses, they only had to cripple one animal to stop a chariot. Once a chariot was
stopped, other soldiers surrounded it and killed the riders. On that day Yue Fei
scored a military victory which lives today in history and legend.

From this short story, you can see that the shield could have various uses in
ancient times. Next, we will list a few shield designs for your reference.

Side Shield (Pang Pai, 旁牌) (Figure 6-3). The large rectangular side shield
was commonly used by foot soldiers to block projectiles, such as arrows, spears,
stones, etc. This kind of side shield was very heavy and large. Its defensive capability was high. However, due to its weight, this kind of shield would lose effectiveness when there was hand-to-hand combat. Therefore, once the enemy had
closed in to the range of hand-to-hand battle, a smaller and lighter shield would
be used immediately. The material used for the side shield was normally wood,
covered with leather.[4]

Leaning Shield (Ai Pai, 挨牌) (Figure 6-4). The leaning shield was also commonly used by foot soldiers. It was heavy and large. According to the available

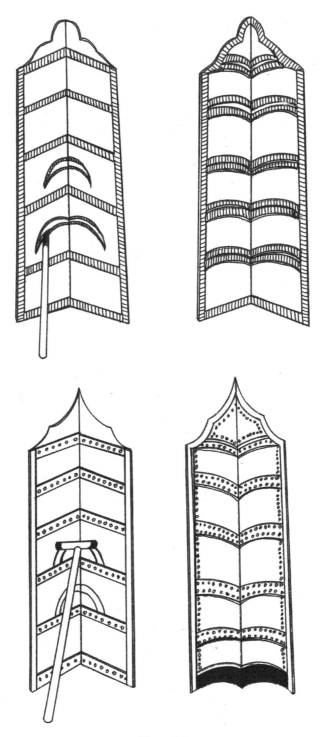

Figure 6-3

documentation, it was made from the wood of the white willow tree. The length was 5 Chi (尺), and the width was 1.5 Chi. The top of the shield was slightly smaller than the bottom. The ropes were used to tighten the entire structure together.[5]

Hand Shield (Shou Pai, 手牌) (Figure 6-5). The hand shield was very similar to the side shield and the leaning shield. Its purpose was also the same. However, its structure was different. The material used for the hand shield was either white willow wood or pine. These woods were light and strong. The length of the hand shield was 5.7 Chi, however, the width was much narrower than both the side shield and the leaning shield, only 1 Chi. The width of the center area of the hand shield was smaller than that of both ends. Therefore, it was lighter and easier to carry for a single soldier over long distances.[6]

Swallow Tail Shield (Yan Wei Pai, 燕尾牌) (Figure 6-6). The swallow tail shield was again very similar to the above three shields, and its purpose was also the same. The main difference for this shield was that it was even narrower than the hand shield, less than 1 Chi. Therefore, it was even lighter than the hand shield, and could be carried and moved faster than any other large shield. Normally, the material used to make the swallow tail shield was a special kind of tree called *Aleurites cordata* (Tong Mu, 桐木). However, because it was narrower, the soldier needed to hide behind the shield with his body turned to the side whenever it was used.[7]

Rattan Shield (Teng Pai, 藤牌) (Figure 6-7). The rattan shield was made from a vine, rattan, that was light and strong. The rattan shield could be used by both foot soldiers and cavalry. Because rattan was grown in the south of China, it therefore became a common material for shields. Also, because there are more

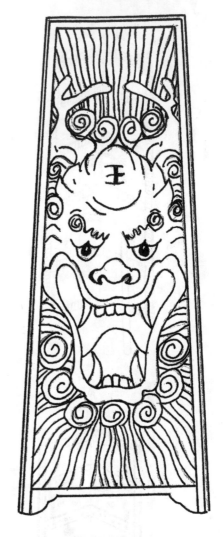

Figure 6-4

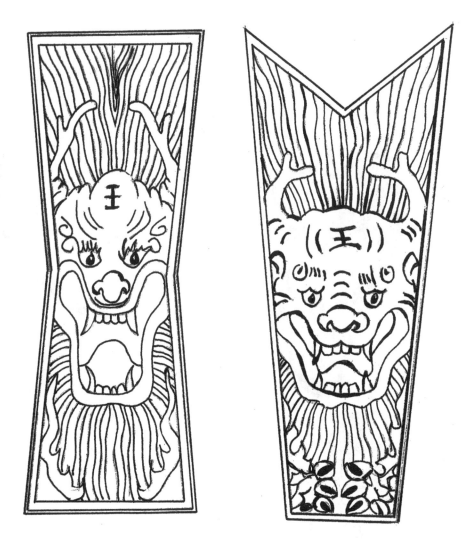

Figure 6-5   Figure 6-6

lakes and rivers in southern China, fewer cavalry units existed. It was therefore used more for foot soldiers than for cavalry.[3]

Cavalry Side Shield (Ji Bing Pang Pai, 騎兵旁牌) (Figure 6-8). The main concerns for constructing a shield for cavalry were weight, size and strength, so that soldiers on horseback were able to move easily. The cavalry side shield was round, so that it could be moved easily on horseback. Moreover, the material was wood, covered with leather. Later, when metallurgical technology advanced to a higher level, a stronger metal shield was developed.

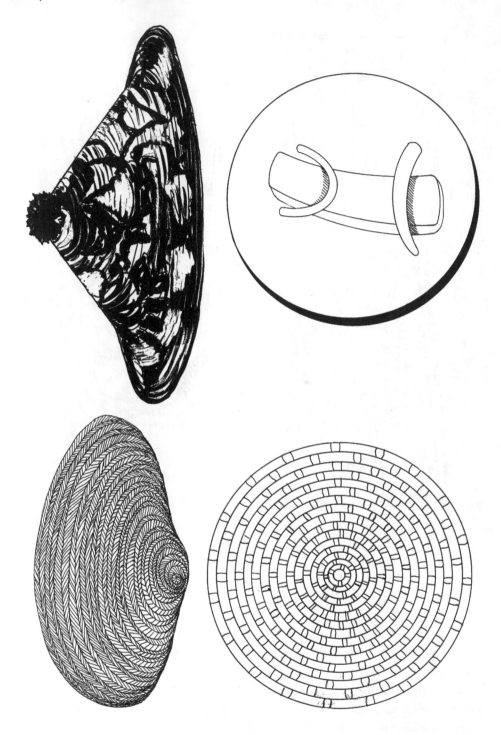

Figure 6-7

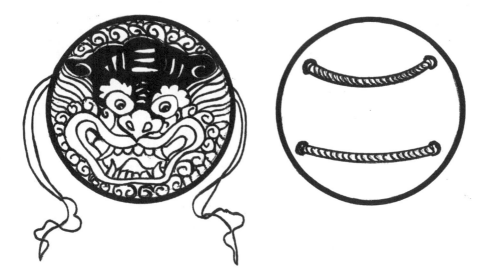

Figure 6-8

6-3. ARMOR

Armor was commonly called "Jia" (shell, 甲) or "Rong Yi" (army clothes, 戎衣) and was designed mainly to protect the body from an enemy's weapon. It was called Jia because, when you are wearing it, it feels like you are protected by a shell. Commonly there are four parts: the helmet (Zhou, 胄 or Dou Jian, 兜鍪), the shoulder and upper chest cover (Pi Bo, 披膊), chest armor (Xiong Kai, 胸鎧), and the leg skirt (Tui Qun, 腿裙).

Armor had different names according to the different dynasties or periods in China. For example, it was called "Long Jia" (Dragon Armor, 龍甲) in South-North Dynasties (420-589 A.D., 南北朝), and He Jia (合甲), or Zhong Jia (衷甲) in the Zhou Dynasty (909-255 B.C., 周朝).[3] Normally, armor for generals or high ranking officers was made from male (犀) and female rhinoceros hide (Si, 兕). Moreover, chest armor was commonly made from a piece of metal.

Next, let us explain the three parts of armor.

Armor (Kai Jia, 鎧甲)

In order to have better mobility in battle, armor was usually made in several pieces (Figure 6-9). If the armor was constructed from a single piece, it would be harder to move the body. Normally, armor includes three parts:

Helmet (Zhou, 胄) (Xiang Dun Mou Tou, 項頓鍪頭) (Dou Jian, 兜鍪) (Figure 6-10). The helmet was used to protect the head and often also the neck. The common material used for the helmet was either leather or metal. While the head area was constructed from a sole piece of leather or metal, the neck area was

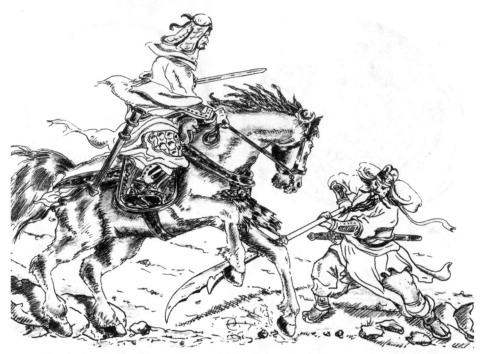

Figure 6-9

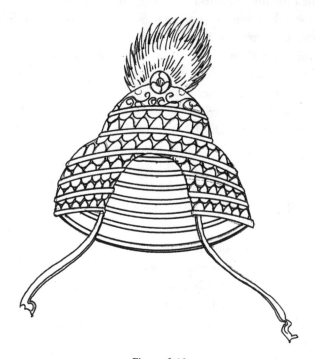

Figure 6-10

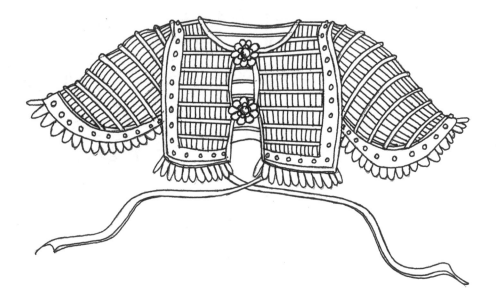

Figure 6-11

constructed from long strips of leather, or chain metal. To avoid the helmet dropping off from the constant movement of battle, two chin straps were used.

Shoulder and Upper Chest Cover (Pi Bo, 披膊) (Figures 6-11 and 6-12). Shoulder cover armor was constructed either from strong leather or less commonly from rhinoceros hide. The shoulder cover was designed to protect the shoulder, upper arms, and upper chest. Again, there were two straps that were used to tighten up the armor.

The material for the upper chest cover armor was the same as the shoulder cover armor. The major purpose of the chest cover armor was to protect the side of the chest area. Again, there were two straps that could be used to tighten it up on the body.

Body Armor (Shen Jia, 身甲) (Figure 6-13). Body armor includes "Chest Armor" (Xiong Kai, 胸鎧) and "Leg Skirt" (Tui Qun, 腿裙). Chest armor was made from a piece of metal, or from the skin of the rhinoceros. There were several pairs of straps which could be used to tighten it firmly on the neck, waist, and upper chest. With body armor, protection of the solar plexus and the groin area was provided.

The leg skirt was two pieces of leather covering, made from leather or rhinoceros hide. Often, the leg skirt covered only the thighs, but it was not uncommon for the skirt to cover the calf.

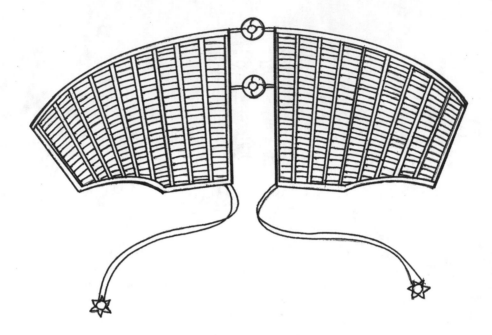

Figure 6-12

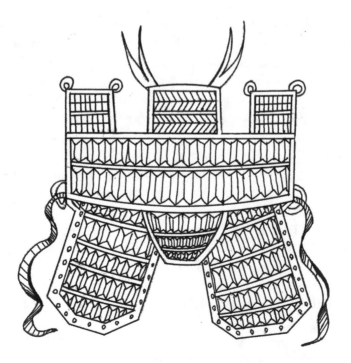

Figure 6-13

If you were to wear all of the armor listed here, equipped from the head to the thighs, it would be very heavy. The main concerns in the design were strength, weight and protection versus mobility. Because weapons were also very heavy, the strength and the endurance of a soldier were usually an important goal of martial training.

References

1. 漢楊雄《方言》卷九：〝盾自關而東或謂之干。〞

2. 唐顏師古《注》：〝盾一名瞂，亦謂之干，即今之旁牌也。〞

3. 戚繼光《紀效新書》卷十一：〝以籐爲牌，近出福建。統子雖不能御格，而矢石槍刀皆少敝，所以代甲冑之用，…。〞

4. 見明茅元儀《武備志》卷一四零〝軍資乘‧器械〞。

5. 明茅元儀《武備志》卷一四零〝軍資乘‧器械〞：〝挨牌亦用白楊木爲之，每面長五尺，闊一尺五寸，上頭比下略小四五分，俱小尺，用繩索乃木橛欖挽之。〞

6. 明茅元儀《武備志》卷一四零〝軍資乘‧器械〞：〝手牌宜用白楊木或松木爲之，取其輕而堅也，長五尺七寸，闊一尺，上下兩頭比中間闊三四分，俱小尺。〞

7. 明茅元儀《武備志》卷一四零〝軍資乘‧器械〞：〝燕尾牌廣中狼柳兵用之，其長與手牌相似，但闊而不滿尺，背如鯽魚，故側身前遍，雖當利刃而不能斷其體輕，故運如鳥翼，而一切矢石皆可避，以按木桐木爲之。〞

8. 南朝徐陵《徐孝穆集‧梁貞陽侯重與王太尉書》：〝霜戈雪戟，無非武庫之兵；龍甲犀渠，皆是雲台之仗。〞

9. 《周禮‧考工記》：〝合甲五屬。〞鄭玄《注》：〝合甲，削革裹肉，但取其表，合以爲甲。〞又〝合甲壽三百年。〞清江永《周禮疑義舉要》：〝犀甲兕甲皆單而不合，合則一甲有兩甲之力，費功多而僧重。〞

10. 《左傳》：魯襄公二十七年：〝辛巳，將盟于宋西門外，楚人衷甲。〞《注》：〝甲在衣中。〞《后漢書‧董卓傳》：〝〔李〕肅以戟刺之，卓衷甲不入，傷臂墜卓。〞

121

CHAPTER 7

Conclusion

結語

Hopefully, this book has served as a basic introduction to ancient Chinese martial weapons and their relationship to the history of China. Detailing the structure or techniques of each of the thousands of weapons used over the course of 50 centuries remains an impossible task, because of the sheer number of weapons and the scarcity of documentation.

This book has attempted to offer you as complete a compilation of ancient Chinese weapons as possible. There were countless weapons developed in each individual martial style in China which have never been documented. This book should serve you as only the first step in such a compilation. I hope that someday other authors can add to the body of knowledge we have regarding these ancient and elegant works of art.

Tables of Weapons

LONG WEAPONS 長兵器

SHORT WEAPONS 短兵器

Very Short Weapons

Short Weapons

SOFT WEAPONS 軟兵器

PROJECTILE AND THROWING WEAPONS 投射兵器

SHIELDS AND ARMOR 盾牌與鎧甲

Shields 盾牌

    1. Side Shield (Pang Pai, 旁牌), p. 112

    2. Leaning Shield (Ai Pai, 挨牌), p. 112

    3. Hand Shield (Shou Pai, 手牌), p. 114

    4. Swallow Tail Shield (Yan Wei Pai, 燕尾牌), p. 114

    5. Rattan Shield (Teng Pai, 籐牌), p. 114

    6. Cavalry Side Shield (Ji Bing Pang Pai, 騎兵旁牌), p. 115

Armor 鎧甲

    1. Armor (Kai Jia, 鎧甲)

        A. Helmet (Zhou, 冑) (Xiang Dun Mou Tou, 項頓鍪頭)

           (Dou Jian, 兜鞬), p. 117

        B. Shoulder and Upper Chest Cover (Pi Bo, 披膊), p. 119

        C. Body Armor (Shen Jia, 身甲), p. 119

Time Table of Chinese History

CHINESE	ENGLISH TRANSLATION	DURATION
五帝紀	The Age of the Five Rulers	(647 Years) 2852-2205 B.C.
夏紀	The Xia Dynasty	(439 Years) 2205-1766 B.C.
商紀（殷紀）	The Shang Dynasty (or Yin Dynasty)	(644 Years) 1766-1122 B.C.
周紀	The Zhou Dynasty	(867 Years) 1122-255 B.C.
秦紀	The Qin dynasty	(49 Years) 255-206 B.C.
漢紀（前漢）（西漢）	The Han Dynasty (Former Han or Western Han)	(231 Years) 206 B.C.-25 A.D.
後漢紀	The Later Han Dynasty (Eastern Han)	(196 Years) 25-221 A.D.
三國	Epoch of The Three Kingdoms	(44 Years) 221-265 A.D.
I. 蜀漢紀	The Minor Han Dynasty	(44 Years) 221-265 A.D.
II. 魏紀	The Wei Dynasty	(45 Years) 220-265 A.D.
III. 吳紀	The Wu Dynasty	(56 Years) 222-278 A.D.
西晉紀	The Western Jin Dynasty	(52 Years) 265-317 A.D.
東晉紀	The Eastern Jin Dynasty	(103 Years) 317-420 A.D.
南北朝	Epoch of Division Between North and South	(169 Years) 420-589 A.D.
劉宋紀	The Song Dynasty (House of Liu)	(59 Years) 420-479 A.D.
北魏紀	The Northern Wei Dynasty (House of Toba)	(149 Years) 386-535 A.D.
西魏紀	The Western Wei Dynasty	(22 Years) 535-557 A.D.
東魏紀	The Eastern Wei Dynasty	(16 Years) 534-550 A.D.
北齊紀	The Northern Qi Dynasty	(39 Years) 550-589 A.D.
北周紀	The Northern Zhou Dynasty	(32 Years) 557-589 A.D.
齊紀	The Qi Dynasty	(23 Years) 479-502 A.D.
梁紀	The Liang Dynasty	(55 Years) 502-557 A.D.
陳紀	The Chen Dynasty	(32 Years) 557-589 A.D.
隋紀	The Sui Dynasty	(29 Years) 589-618 A.D.
唐紀	The Tang Dynasty	(389 Years) 618-907 A.D.

五代	The Epoch of the Five Dynasties	(53 Years) 907-960 A.D.
後梁紀	The Posterior Liang Dynasty	(16 Years) 907-923 A.D.
後唐紀	The Posterior Tang Dynasty	(13 Years) 923-936 A.D.
後晉紀	The Posterior Jin Dynasty	(11 Years) 936-947 A.D.
後漢紀	The Posterior Han Dynasty	(4 Years) 947-951 A.D.
後周紀	The Posterior Zhou Dynasty	(9 Years) 951-960 A.D.
遼紀	The Liao Dynasty (Khitan Tartars)	(218 Years) 907-1125 A.D.
西遼紀	The Western Liao Dynasty (Khitan Tartars)	(43 Years) 1125-1169 A.D.
宋紀	The Song Dynasty	(167 Years) 960-1127 A.D.
南宋紀	The Southern Song Dynasty	(153 Years) 1127-1280 A.D.
金紀	The Jin Dynasty (Niu Zhen Tartars)	(145 Years) 1115-1260 A.D.
元紀	The Yuan Dynasty (Mongols)	(162 Years) 1206-1368 A.D.
明紀	The Ming Dynasty	(276 Years) 1368-1644 A.D.
清紀	The Qing Dynasty	(268 Years) 1644-1912 A.D.
中華民國	The Republic of China	1912 -

Translation and Glossary of Chinese Terms

Bai He 白鶴
Means "White Crane." One of the southern Chinese martial styles.

Bai La Gan 白臘桿
White wax wood, which only grows in Northern China.

Bing 兵
Soldiers. Bing is also commonly used as an abbreviation of Bingqi (martial weapons).

Bingqi 兵器
Martial weapons.

Canton (Guangdong) 廣東
A province in southern China.

Cao-Cao 曹操
The ruler of Wei. Wei was one of the three kingdoms in The Three Kingdoms Dynasty which followed the Han Dynasty and lasted 60 years (220-280 A.D.).

Chang Bing 長兵
Means "long weapons."

Chang Chuan (Changquan) 長拳
Means "Long Range Fist." Chang Chuan includes all northern Chinese long range martial styles.

Chang Jiang (Yangtze River) 長江 〔揚子江〕
Literally, long river. Refers to the Yangtze river in southern China.

Changquan (Chang Chuan) 長拳
Means "Long Range Fist." Changquan includes all northern Chinese long range martial styles.

Cheng, Gin-Gsao 曾金灶
Dr. Yang, Jwing-Ming's White Crane master.

Chi Kung (Qigong) 氣功
The Gongfu of Qi, which means the study of Qi.

Chi You 蚩尤
The opponent of the Yellow Emperor (Huang Di) during the years 2697-2597 B.C.

Chi 尺
Ancient Chinese units of length (1 Chi=0.3581 meters).

Chin Na (Qin Na) 擒拿

Literally means "grab control." A component of Chinese martial arts which emphasizes grabbing techniques, to control your opponent's joints, in conjunction with attacking certain acupuncture cavities.

Da Mo 達摩

The Indian Buddhist monk who is credited with creating the *Yi Jin Jing* and *Xi Sui Jing* while at the Shaolin monastery around 527 A.D. His last name was Sardili and he was also known as Bodhidarma. He was once the prince of a small tribe in southern India.

Da Yong 大庸

A county of Hunan Province.

Dian Xue Massages 點穴按摩

Chinese massage techniques in which the acupuncture cavities are stimulated through pressing. Dian Xue massage is also called acupressure, and is the root of Japanese Shiatsu.

Duan Bing 短兵

Means "short weapons."

Fujian Province 短兵

A province located in southeast China.

Gan Jiang 干將

A very famous sword maker, who also named one of his best swords "Gan Jiang." His wife, Mo Xie was also a well-known sword maker at the time.

Gong (Kung) 功

Energy or hard work.

Gongfu (Kung Fu) 功夫

Means "energy-time." Anything which will take time and energy to learn or to accomplish is called Gongfu.

Guai Zi Ma 拐子馬

An ancient version of the tank created by the Jin commander Wu Zhu during the Chinese Southern Song Dynasty (1127-1280 A.D.) It was a chariot carrying armored men, drawn by three fully armored horses which were connected by a chain. It was extremely difficult to disable either the horses or the riders, and so they completely dominated the battlefield.

Guan Dao 關刀

The Guan Dao was created in the Chinese Three Kingdoms Period (221-280 A.D.) and was used by Guan Yu (or Guan, Yun-Chang). This Long-Handled Saber was also called "Green-Dragon Scything-Moon Saber," (Qing Long Yan Yue Dao) or simply "Green Dragon Saber" (Qing Long Dao)

Guan Yu (or Guan, Yun-Chang) 關羽、關雲長

A Chinese hero during the Chinese Three Kingdoms Period (221-280 A.D.).

Guangdong province 廣東省

A province located in southeast China.

Guoshu (Wushu) 國術〔武術〕

Abbreviation of "Zhongguo Wushu," which means "Chinese Martial Techniques."

Hainan Island 海南島

An island in the South of Guangdong Province. Hainan Island belongs to Guangdong (i.e., Canton) Province.

Han 漢
A Dynasty in Chinese history (206 B.C.-221 A.D.).

Han 漢族
The major race in China.

Han, Ching-Tang 韓慶堂
A well known Chinese martial artist, especially in Taiwan in the last forty years. Master Han is also Dr. Yang, Jwing-Ming's Long Fist Grand Master.

He Lu 闔閭
A Wu emperor who loved collecting sword.

Henan 河南省
The province in China where the Shaolin Temple is located.

Hu Shou 護手
The hand protection for the weapon-hand (hand holding the weapon).

Huang Di (2690-2590 B.C.) 黃帝
Huang Di, called the "Yellow Emperor" because he occupied the territory near the Yellow River.

Hunan Province 湖南省
A province near the middle of China.

Ji, Long-Feng 姬隆丰
The creator of the Xin-Yi martial style.

Jian Chi 劍池
Sword Pond. Located in Suzhou of Jiangsu Province.

Jiangxi Province 江西
A province of China.

Jin, Shao-Feng 金紹峰
Dr. Yang, Jwing-Ming's White Crane grand master.

Ju Que 巨闕
One of the famous swords forged by Ou Ye Zi, during the Chinese Spring and Autumn Period (722-484 B.C.), and the Warring States Period (403-222 B.C.). It is said that this sword was so sharp that if dipped in water, it would be withdrawn perfectly dry.

Kao Tao 高濤
Master Yang, Jwing-Ming's first Taijiquan master.

Kung (Gong) 功
Means energy or hard work.

Kung Fu (Gongfu) 功夫
Means "energy-time." Anything which will take time and energy to learn or to accomplish is called Kung Fu.

Li 黎族
A tribe on the Hainan Island of Guangdong Province.

Li, Mao-Ching 李茂清
Dr. Yang, Jwing-Ming's Long Fist master.

Li, Tai Bai 李太白
A famous poet in the Tang Dynasty (618-907 A.D.).

Liu Bei 劉備
The ruler of Han. Han was one of the three kingdoms in The Three Kingdoms Dynasty.

Long Quan 龍泉
A county in Zhejiang Province which is well known for producing good weapons.

Lu Bu 呂布
A well known general during the Chinese Three Kingdoms era (220-265 A.D.).

Luoyang 洛陽
A city in Henan Province.

Mo Xie 莫邪
A very famous sword maker, who named one of her best swords "Mo Xie." Her Husband, Gan Jiang was also a well-known sword maker at the time.

Ou Ye Zi 歐冶子
One of the three most famous sword makers in the Chinese Spring and Autumn Period (722-484 B.C.) and the Warring States Period (403-222 B.C.). The other two well-known sword makers were Gan Jiang and Mo Xie. Ou Ye Zi forged two very famous swords, Ju Que and Zhan Lu.

Pu Yuan 蒲元
A famous sword maker during the Chinese Three Kingdoms Period (221-280 A.D.).

Qi (Chi) 氣
Chinese term for universal energy. A current popular model is that the Qi circulating in the human body is bioelectric in nature.

Qi Mei Gun 齊眉棍
Equal Eyebrows Rod. Name of the southern staff with a length equal to the height of a martial artist, from his/her feet to their eyebrow. Qi Mei Gun is also the name of a staff sequence.

Qi, Ji-Guang 戚繼光
A well known general in the Ming Dynasty (1386-1644 A.D.).

Qigong (Chi Kung) 氣功
The Gongfu of Qi, which means the study of Qi.

Qin (Chin) 擒
Means 'to catch" or "to seize."

Qin Na (Chin Na) 擒拿
Literally means "grab control." A component of Chinese martial arts which emphasizes grabbing techniques to control your opponent's joints, in conjunction with attacking certain acupuncture cavities.

Qin Shi 秦始皇
An emperor of the Qin Dynasty (255-206 B.C.).

Qin Yang 沁陽
A county in Henan Province.

Qing Long Dao 青龍刀
Green Dragon Saber. Name of a long handled sable used by Guan Yu during the Chinese Three Kingdoms era (220-265 A.D.). It was also called "Green-Dragon Scything-Moon Saber."

Rong 戎人
A tribe in ancient western China.

San Xi Province 山西省
A province of China.

Shaolin 少林
"Young woods." Name of the Shaolin Temple.

Shaolin Temple 少林寺
A monastery located in Henan Province, China. The Shaolin Temple is well known because of its martial arts training.

Shi Ba Ban Wu Qi 十八般武器
Eighteen Representative Weapons. The specific weapons changed from dynasty to dynasty. Shi Ba Ban Wu Qi implies all of the weapons.

Shu 蜀
Sichuan Province is also called Shu.

Si 兕
A female rhinoceros.

Si Ming Mountain 四明山
A mountain in Zhejiang Province.

Sichuan Province (Shu) 四川省〔蜀〕
A province in western China.

Song Taizu 宋太祖
A Song emperor, at the beginning of the Song Dynasty (960 A.D.).

Sun Quan 孫權
The ruler of Wu. Wu was one of the three kingdoms in the era of the Three Kingdoms Dynasty.

Sun, Yat-Sen 孫中山
The father of China. He is credited with leading the revolt against the Qing Dynasty in 1911 A.D., and for attempting to introduce democratic reforms into China's political system.

Sun Bin 孫臏
A well-known martial artist and military strategist during the Chinese Spring and Autumn Period and the Warring States Period (722-222 B.C.).

Suzhou 蘇州
A city in Jiangsu Province.

Tai Chi Chuan (Taijiquan) 太極拳
A Chinese internal martial style which is based on the theory of Taiji (grand ultimate).

Taiji 太極
Means "grand ultimate." It is this force which generates two poles, Yin and Yang.

Taijiquan (Tai Chi Chuan) 太極拳
A Chinese internal martial style which is based on the theory of Taiji (grand ultimate).

Taipei 台北
The capital city of Taiwan, located in the north.

Taiwan 台灣
An island to the south-east of mainland China. Also known as "Formosa."

Taiwan University 台灣大學
A well known university located in northern Taiwan.

Taizuquan 太祖拳
A style of Chinese external martial arts.

Tamkang 淡江
Name of a University in Taiwan.

Tamkang College Guoshu Club 淡江國術社
A Chinese martial arts club founded by Dr. Yang when he was studying in Tamkang College.

Teng 藤
Rattan.

Teng Pai Jun 藤牌軍
Name of the rattan shield army created by Marshal Yue Fei to fight against Guai Zi Ma.

Tong Mu 桐木
A special kind of tree called *Aleurites cordata*. The wood from the tree was commonly used for weapons manufacture in ancient times.

Tui Na 推拿
Push and grab. A Chinese Qigong massage technique for healing.

Tung oil 桐油
Wood-oil obtained from the seeds of paulownia.

Wen Jian 文劍
Scholar sword. The scholar sword, also known as the female sword (Ci Jian), is lighter and shorter than the martial or male sword (Xiong Jian).

Wilson Chen 陳威伸
Dr. Yang, Jwing-Ming's friend.

Wu 武
Means "martial."

Wu Jian 武劍
Martial sword. The martial sword, also known as the male sword (Xiong Jian), is heavier and longer than the scholar or female sword (Ci Jian).

Wu Kang 武康
A county in Zhejiang Province known for the production of high quality ancient weapons.

Wushu 武術
Literally, "martial techniques."

Wuyi 武藝
Literally, "martial arts."

Wu Zhu 兀朮

The Jin commander who created the terrifying weapon "Guai Zi Ma." The Guai Zi Ma was an ancient version of the tank. It was a chariot carrying armored men, drawn by three fully armored horses which were connected by a chain. It was extremely difficult to disable either the horses or the riders, and so they completely dominated the battlefield.

Wuqi 武器

Literally translates as "martial instruments" or "martial weapons."

Wushu (Gongfu) 武術〔功夫〕

Literally, martial technique. It is commonly called Guoshu (i.e., country techniques) in Taiwan or Gongfu in the western society.

Xi 犀

A male rhinoceros.

Xin-Yin style 心意門

A martial style created by Ji, Long-Feng.

Xing Yuan 性圓

Name of a Buddhist monk. According to legend, during the Northern Song Dynasty (960-1127 A.D.), he traveled to Tibet and learned the techniques of the dart, later bringing the weapon back to China.

Xinzhu Xian 新竹縣

Birthplace of Dr. Yang, Jwing-Ming in Taiwan.

Xiou Gang 蕭綱

Name of an author who wrote a book about the Shuo techniques, used in horse back fighting, during Liang Jian Wen era (550-551 A.D.).

Xiyu 西域

The territory on the Western side of China.

Xu, Liang-Chen 徐亮臣

Name of a person who created many new weapons during the Northern Song Dynasty (960-1127 A.D.).

Xuan Niu 玄女

Huang Di's great-great-granddaughter.

Xue Dang 血擋

Blood Stopper. A special type of tassel made from the hair of the horse tail. This tassel is tied near the spear head to stop blood from flowing onto the staff, which might affect the skillful use of the spear.

Yang, Jwing-Ming 楊俊敏

Author of this book.

Yang Xie 楊偕

A general during the Song Ren Zong era (1023-1064 A.D.).

Yangtze River 揚子江

Also called Chang Jiang (i.e., long river). One of the two major rivers in China.

Yi Jin Jing 易筋經

Literally, *Changing Muscle/Tendon Classic,* usually called *The Muscle/Tendon Changing Classic.* Credited to Da Mo around 550 A.D., this book discusses Wai Dan Qigong training for strengthening the physical body.

Yue Fei 岳飛

A Chinese hero in the Southern Song Dynasty (1127-1279 A.D.). Said to have created Ba Duan Jin, Xingyiquan and Yue's Ying Zhua.

Zhan Lu 湛盧

One of the two famous swords made by sword maker Ou Ye Zi, during the Chinese Spring and Autumn Period (722-484 B.C.) and the Warring States Period (403-222 B.C.). The other sword was called "Ju Que."

Zhang, Xiang-San 張詳三

A well known Chinese martial artist in Taiwan.

Zhong Guo 中國

Literally, "central country." This name was given to China by its neighboring countries. China was considered the cultural and spiritual center of Asia in ancient times.

Zhejiang Province 浙江省

A province of China near the south-east coast.

Zhuo Lu 涿鹿

Location of an ancient battle between the Emperor Huang Di's forces and his opponent, Chi You.

Index

101 REFLECTIONS ON TAI CHI CHUAN
108 INSIGHTS INTO TAI CHI CHUAN
A SUDDEN DAWN: THE EPIC JOURNEY OF BODHIDHARMA
A WOMAN'S QIGONG GUIDE
ADVANCING IN TAE KWON DO
ANALYSIS OF SHAOLIN CHIN NA 2ND ED
ANCIENT CHINESE WEAPONS
THE ART AND SCIENCE OF STAFF FIGHTING
THE ART AND SCIENCE OF STICK FIGHTING
ART OF HOJO UNDO
ARTHRITIS RELIEF, 3D ED.
BACK PAIN RELIEF, 2ND ED.
BAGUAZHANG, 2ND ED.
BRAIN FITNESS
CARDIO KICKBOXING ELITE
CHIN NA IN GROUND FIGHTING
CHINESE FAST WRESTLING
CHINESE FITNESS
CHINESE TUI NA MASSAGE
CHOJUN
COMPLETE MARTIAL ARTIST
COMPREHENSIVE APPLICATIONS OF SHAOLIN CHIN NA
CONFLICT COMMUNICATION
CROCODILE AND THE CRANE: A NOVEL
CUTTING SEASON: A XENON PEARL MARTIAL ARTS THRILLER
DAO DE JING
DAO IN ACTION
DEFENSIVE TACTICS
DESHI: A CONNOR BURKE MARTIAL ARTS THRILLER
DIRTY GROUND
DR. WU'S HEAD MASSAGE
DUKKHA HUNGRY GHOSTS
DUKKHA REVERB
DUKKHA, THE SUFFERING: AN EYE FOR AN EYE
DUKKHA UNLOADED
ENZAN: THE FAR MOUNTAIN, A CONNOR BURKE MARTIAL ARTS
    THRILLER
ESSENCE OF SHAOLIN WHITE CRANE
EVEN IF IT KILLS ME
EXPLORING TAI CHI
FACING VIOLENCE
FIGHT BACK
FIGHT LIKE A PHYSICIST
THE FIGHTER'S BODY
FIGHTER'S FACT BOOK
FIGHTER'S FACT BOOK 2
THE FIGHTING ARTS
FIGHTING THE PAIN RESISTANT ATTACKER
FIRST DEFENSE
FORCE DECISIONS: A CITIZENS GUIDE
FOX BORROWS THE TIGER'S AWE
INSIDE TAI CHI
THE JUDO ADVANTAGE
THE JUJI GATAME ENCYCLOPEDIA
KAGE: THE SHADOW, A CONNOR BURKE MARTIAL ARTS THRILLER
KARATE SCIENCE
KATA AND THE TRANSMISSION OF KNOWLEDGE
KRAV MAGA COMBATIVES
KRAV MAGA PROFESSIONAL TACTICS
KRAV MAGA WEAPON DEFENSES
LITTLE BLACK BOOK OF VIOLENCE
LIUHEBAFA FIVE CHARACTER SECRETS
MARTIAL ARTS ATHLETE
MARTIAL ARTS INSTRUCTION
MARTIAL WAY AND ITS VIRTUES
MASK OF THE KING
MEDITATIONS ON VIOLENCE
MERIDIAN QIGONG EXERCISES
MIND/BODY FITNESS
MINDFUL EXERCISE
THE MIND INSIDE TAI CHI
THE MIND INSIDE YANG STYLE TAI CHI CHUAN
MUGAI RYU
NATURAL HEALING WITH QIGONG
NORTHERN SHAOLIN SWORD, 2ND ED.
OKINAWA'S COMPLETE KARATE SYSTEM: ISSHIN RYU
THE PAIN-FREE BACK

PAIN-FREE JOINTS
POWER BODY
PRINCIPLES OF TRADITIONAL CHINESE MEDICINE
THE PROTECTOR ETHIC
QIGONG FOR HEALTH & MARTIAL ARTS 2ND ED.
QIGONG FOR LIVING
QIGONG FOR TREATING COMMON AILMENTS
QIGONG MASSAGE
QIGONG MEDITATION: EMBRYONIC BREATHING
QIGONG MEDITATION: SMALL CIRCULATION
QIGONG, THE SECRET OF YOUTH: DA MO'S CLASSICS
QUIET TEACHER: A XENON PEARL MARTIAL ARTS THRILLER
RAVEN'S WARRIOR
REDEMPTION
ROOT OF CHINESE QIGONG, 2ND ED.
SAMBO ENCYCLOPEDIA
SCALING FORCE
SELF-DEFENSE FOR WOMEN
SENSEI: A CONNOR BURKE MARTIAL ARTS THRILLER
SHIHAN TE: THE BUNKAI OF KATA
SHIN GI TAI: KARATE TRAINING FOR BODY, MIND, AND SPIRIT
SIMPLE CHINESE MEDICINE
SIMPLE QIGONG EXERCISES FOR HEALTH, 3RD ED.
SIMPLIFIED TAI CHI CHUAN, 2ND ED.
SOLO TRAINING
SOLO TRAINING 2
SPOTTING DANGER BEFORE DANGER SPOTS YOU
SUMO FOR MIXED MARTIAL ARTS
SUNRISE TAI CHI
SUNSET TAI CHI
SURVIVING ARMED ASSAULTS
TAE KWON DO: THE KOREAN MARTIAL ART
TAEKWONDO BLACK BELT POOMSAE
TAEKWONDO: A PATH TO EXCELLENCE
TAEKWONDO: ANCIENT WISDOM FOR THE MODERN WARRIOR
TAEKWONDO: DEFENSE AGAINST WEAPONS
TAEKWONDO: SPIRIT AND PRACTICE
TAO OF BIOENERGETICS
TAI CHI BALL QIGONG: FOR HEALTH AND MARTIAL ARTS
TAI CHI BALL WORKOUT FOR BEGINNERS
THE TAI CHI BOOK
TAI CHI CHIN NA: THE SEIZING ART OF TAI CHI CHUAN,
    2ND ED.
TAI CHI CHUAN CLASSICAL YANG STYLE, 2ND ED.
TAI CHI CHUAN MARTIAL POWER, 3RD ED.
TAI CHI CONNECTIONS
TAI CHI DYNAMICS
TAI CHI FOR DEPRESSION
TAI CHI IN 10 WEEKS
TAI CHI QIGONG, 3RD ED.
TAI CHI SECRETS OF THE ANCIENT MASTERS
TAI CHI SECRETS OF THE WU & LI STYLES
TAI CHI SECRETS OF THE WU STYLE
TAI CHI SECRETS OF THE YANG STYLE
TAI CHI SWORD: CLASSICAL YANG STYLE, 2ND ED.
TAI CHI SWORD FOR BEGINNERS
TAI CHI WALKING
TAIJIQUAN THEORY OF DR. YANG, JWING-MING
TAO OF BIOENERGETICS
TENGU: THE MOUNTAIN GOBLIN, A CONNOR BURKE MARTIAL ARTS
    THRILLER
TIMING IN THE FIGHTING ARTS
TRADITIONAL CHINESE HEALTH SECRETS
TRADITIONAL TAEKWONDO
TRAINING FOR SUDDEN VIOLENCE
TRUE WELLNESS
TRUE WELLNESS: THE MIND
TRUE WELLNESS: THE HEART
THE WARRIOR'S MANIFESTO
WAY OF KATA
WAY OF KENDO AND KENJITSU
WAY OF SANCHIN KATA
WAY TO BLACK BELT
WESTERN HERBS FOR MARTIAL ARTISTS
WILD GOOSE QIGONG
WINNING FIGHTS
WISDOM'S WAY
XINGYIQUAN

DVDS FROM YMAA

more products available from . . .

YMAA Publication Center, Inc. 楊氏東方文化出版中心

1-800-669-8892 • info@ymaa.com • www.ymaa.com

Printed in the USA
CPSIA information can be obtained
at www.ICGtesting.com
JSHW060041150824
68134JS00028B/2585